the new art of erotic massage

dr. andrew yorke

photography by john davis

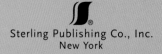

Sterling Publishing Co., Inc.
New York

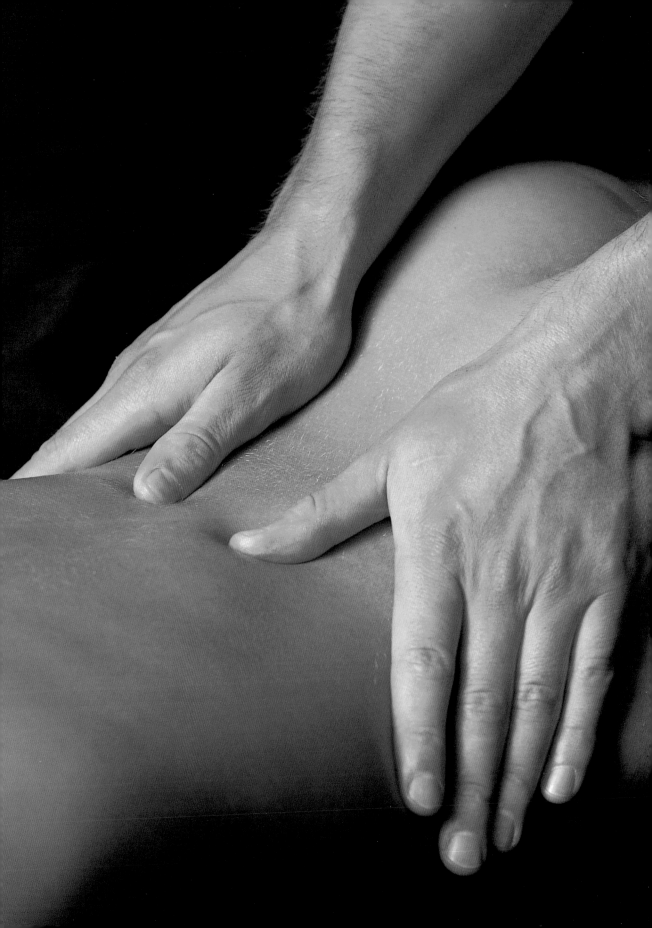

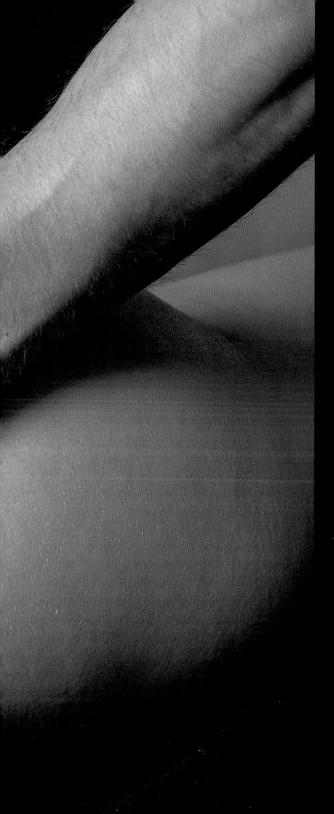

Photography by John Davis
Design by John Round Design
Art Direction by Nigel Wright
Index by Bill Johncocks

Massage should not be considered as a replacement for
professional medical treatment; a physician should be
consulted in all matters relating to health and especially
in relation to any symptoms which may require
diagnosis or medical attention. Care should be taken
during pregnancy, particularly in the use of essential oils
and pressure points. Essential oils should not be
ingested and used for babies and children only on
professional advice.

Library of Congress Cataloging-in-Publication Data
Available

10 9 8 7 6 5 4 3 2 1

Published in 2007 by Sterling Publishing Co., Inc.
387 Park Avenue South, New York, NY 10016

First published in the UK in 1998 by Blandford
This edition first published in the UK in 2007 by Cassell Illustrated
A division of Octopus Publishing Group Ltd.
Copyright © 2007 by Cassell Illustrated
Text copyright © 1998 by Dr. Andrew Yorke

Distributed in Canada by Sterling Publishing
c/o Canadian Manda Group, 165 Dufferin Street,
Toronto, Ontario, Canada M6K 3H6

Printed in China
All rights reserved

Sterling ISBN-13: 978-1-4027-4541-6
          ISBN-10: 1-4027-4541-9

For information about custom editions, special sales,
premium and corporate purchases, please contact Sterling
Special Sales Department at 800-805-5489 or
specialsales@sterlingpub.com.

Contents

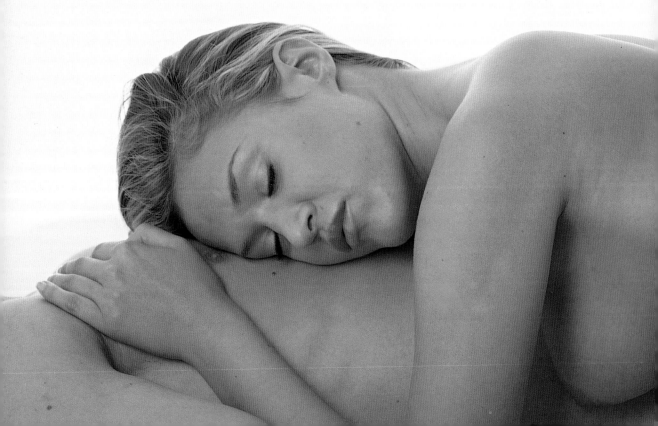

Introduction

Massage is probably one of the oldest and simplest "treatments" known to man. It almost certainly started as simple touching and became more structured and formalized as it was found that people derived benefit from particular types of touch in different situations and conditions.

Massage also has a very distinguished history. Hippocrates, the father of medicine, wrote, "The physician must be experienced in many things, but assuredly in rubbing. . . . For rubbing can bind a joint that is too loose, and loosen one that is too rigid." Pliny, the Roman naturalist, was regularly rubbed to alleviate his asthma, and Julius Caesar, who had epilepsy, was pinched all over each day to relieve neuralgia and headaches.

Eastern cultures have always considered massage to be important and for several thousand years Oriental physicians have used it as a form of healing. Shiatsu, for example, originated from Japanese massage techniques and has been enhanced by ideas gained from acupuncture and even Western techniques such as osteopathy and chiropractic.

In the Middle Ages, however, massage fell from use in Europe, mainly because the Church taught that such pleasures of the flesh hindered an individual's spiritual growth. It wasn't until the beginning of the nineteenth century that a Swede, Per Henrik Ling, developed what we now call Swedish massage— based on his knowledge of gymnastics, and of Greek, Roman, Chinese, and Egyptian techniques. In 1813 the first college offering his form of massage was founded in Stockholm and from this beginning the art and benefits of massage have become known and practiced throughout the Western world.

Today, many people think of massage as a form of "medical" treatment. And indeed it is used to relieve stress, tension and emotional trauma; and to heal damaged muscles and skeletal supporting tissues. But in addition to this it is now increasingly being seen as a means of communication between people who use it as a way of showing love and care, thus enriching interpersonal relationships.

Those who massage one another usually find that their relationship changes for the better. For this reason, therapists such as myself find it useful in helping couples to learn about one another and by doing so to improve their emotional and sexual lives.

Massage today has yet another role to play. At a time when increasing numbers of young couples are delaying intercourse until they are married, or are actually concerned that sexual encounters might threaten their health, some are looking for alternatives to genital penetration. Few people now talk of "safe sex" and most realize that the best one can claim is safer sex, except with a partner whose sexual history is totally known and trustworthy. In this context increasing numbers of couples find that erotic massage, perhaps ending in mutual masturbation, is the only kind of sex that is safe enough or morally acceptable to them until they are ready to settle down with a partner whose sexual history they trust.

It is against this background of changing sexual practices that I have written this book. I hope that it will answer both the needs of those who are not yet in a long-term, stable relationship and want to feel sexually "safe" and of those couples who have been together for many years and want to enrich their sensual and erotic life together.

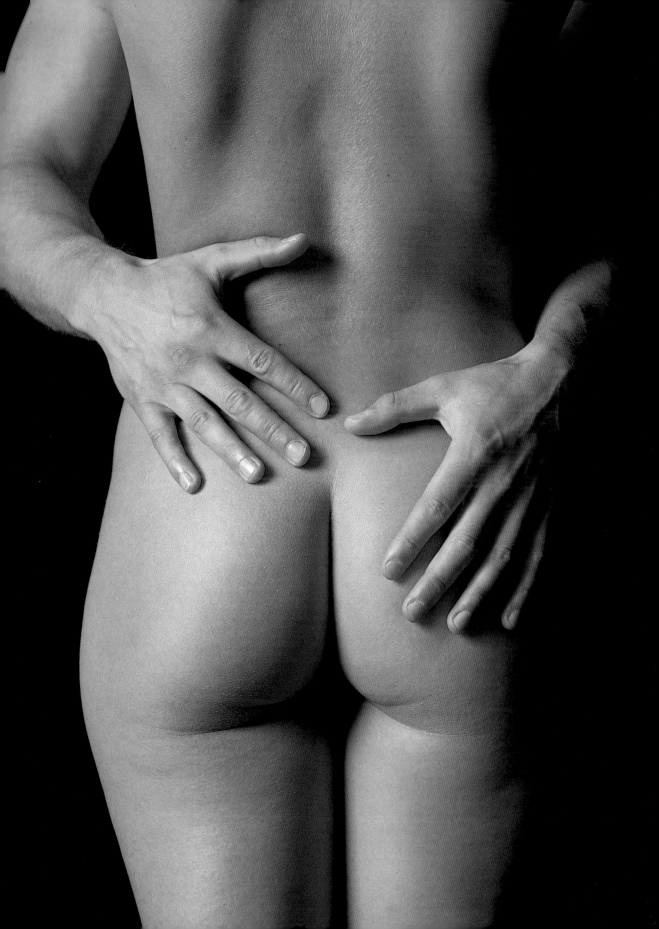

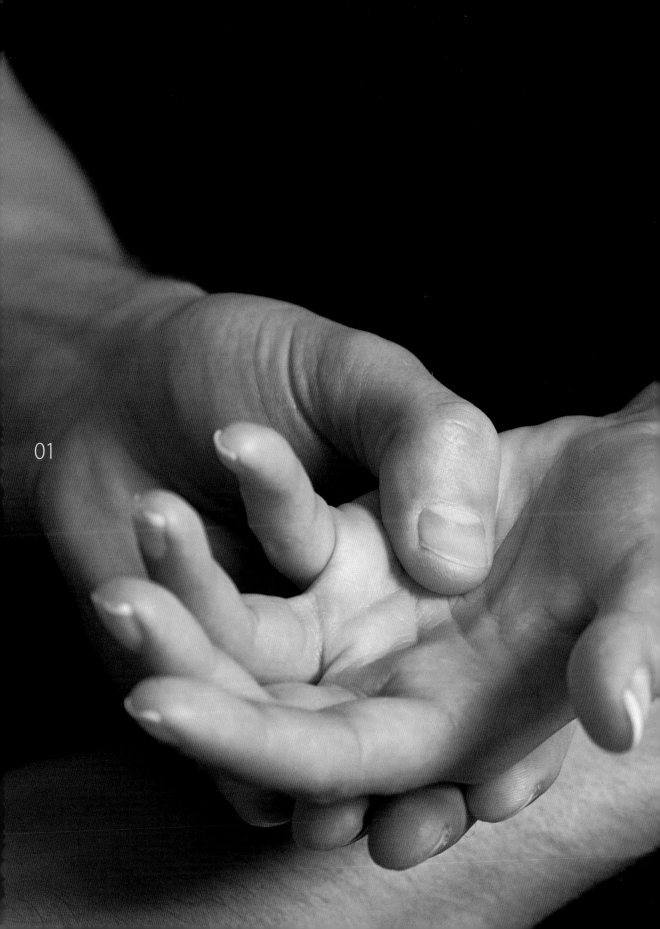

01

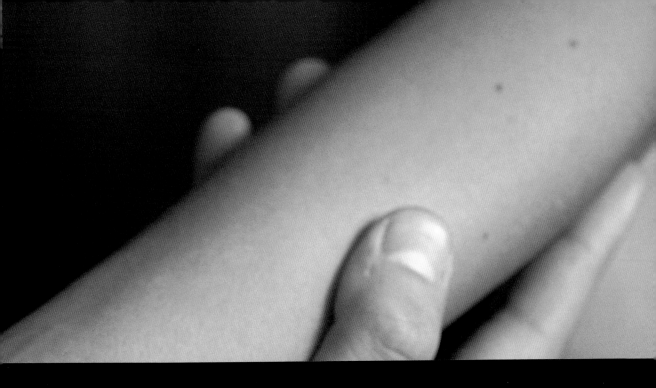

Starting at the beginning

What is massage? Massage is simply a formalized, structured form of touching, so perhaps the place to start is to look at touch and see why it is so vital for human well-being.

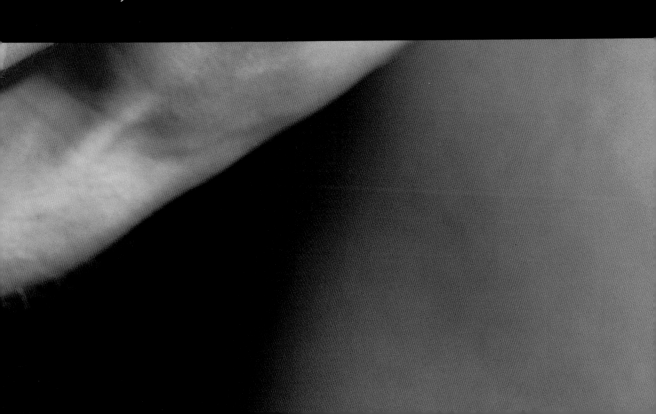

In our so-called permissive society, in which most of our senses are so richly catered for, it is amazing that the sense of touch is ignored. In fact, we live in an almost "no-touch" society. This has come about because, over the centuries, touching others has come to be seen as having a sexual connotation.

Certainly, sex does involve touch but it is quite ridiculous to avoid all touching on the basis that a gesture might lead to sex. Alas, this is exactly what has happened in the Western world. We live in a culture that has many negative views about and prohibitions on sex, and consequently touching has come to be governed by these very same restrictions, as if touching were sex—which, of course, it is not.

Because many of us, once past the cradle or early childhood, touch and are touched so little we understandably find it difficult to touch others in any circumstances—even sexual. I see many couples who have engaged quite happily in all kinds of sexual acts for years but who are intimidated by touching one another because they are unused to that particular form of intimacy. Such people can truly be said to be "out of touch" with their bodies. Indeed, in many men the constant demand for more sex is frequently an unconscious need for touching (and being touched) and closeness. They believe, erroneously, that they should not ask for touching for its own sake and so try to make it "respectable" by including genital activity. After all, in our culture, men aren't supposed to ask for a cuddle or a stroke!

Although no one can be absolutely sure, it appears that touch is the first sense that we develop in the womb. So touch is a primal sensation which, even in adult life, takes us back to our earliest days in the womb. This understandably makes touch very special for human beings. Indeed, the American psychologist S. M. Jourard showed that people's perceptions of how much they were touched were closely related to their sense of personal self-esteem. Most people, when they are prevented from touching and being touched, feel painfully alone and isolated. A US study found that people forbidden skin contact complained of such feelings. Clearly, touch has implications for us that go far beyond making things better when we are ill—the "medical" purpose of massage.

All kinds of pains, emotional or physical, evoke a response that usually involves touching of some kind. When a child falls over the parent lovingly "rubs it better" and holds, kisses and cuddles their child. All of these actions convey to the child that he or she is loved and valued and probably do more good than any number of pills and potions. Doctors and nurses touch their patients, albeit in a somewhat clinical way; healers throughout history have performed the ceremony of the "laying on of hands" and most of us feel we want to touch, hold or cuddle someone we care for when they are distressed or ill.

Touch is a vital communication system that says "I care for you" and whether we are three or ninety-three it unconsciously takes us back to the time when we were babies in our mothers' arms. We feel safe.

Unfortunately, as we grow up we receive less and less in the way of loving, physical contact and boys especially are taught—usually quite unconsciously—by their parents, that they should be tough. They should not need or want cuddling, touching, stroking, or kissing in times of adversity. However, it is a fact that we never outgrow our needs for touch and in today's "nuclear" family we have all too few people who are available to give us such attention even if they were prepared to do so. By and large it is more difficult to accept touch from a stranger and yet members of our own families may have become virtual strangers.

The least stringent anti-touch taboo is between mothers and their daughters—because they are of the same sex and it is accepted in our culture that women are by nature more emotional and caring. As a result, women fare better in adult life, being far more willing, and able, to touch one another nonsexually without feeling bad about it. Men, in contrast, can be almost phobic on the subject. Men will cuddle and caress babies, because they are said to be "asexual." However, as their children begin to grow up and develop more clearly defined "sexual identities," some men become increasingly ill at ease in touching them at all, for fear of being seen as sexually provocative. It depresses me to hear fathers saying that they fear cuddling their own children lest they be accused of unhealthy motives. And heterosexual adult men almost never touch one another if they can help it.

This does not mean that men cease to need to be touched; rather that they find ways that are culturally sanctioned to satisfy their needs. This they do in a sexual relationship with their partner and in sporting activities where touching is permitted.

However, as much as we try to fool ourselves, touch is so basic to our human condition that we all try to get it in whatever way we can. For example, many women who do not have a satisfying relationship with their husbands say that touching and cuddling their babies and children helps to compensate for lack of such contact in their adult relationship. Indeed, it is my professional experience that some women have more children in order to hold on to the closeness of physical touching and togetherness when their earlier offspring become more independent.

Ashley Montagu, in his book *Touching: The Human Significance of the Skin* (1971), maintains that the basic need to be touched must be satisfied if the organism is to survive. The distinguished psychologist Alexander Lowen feels that schizophrenia may come about as a result of too little touching in early life. The schizophrenic is seen as being "out of touch" with himself. There are also studies that show links between touch deprivation in childhood and later violence.

Even this brief review of the importance of touch must convince the reader that human beings were indeed made to touch and to be touched. If this were not so, it would be unlikely that such a great proportion of our brains would be devoted to the sense of touch.

So, in answer to the question "what is massage?"— it is simply a systematic form of touching that produces various predictable results. Let us now look more closely at the different types of massage.

Types of massage
Over the centuries, many forms of massage have been developed as methods of healing. They include:

Aromatherapy in which essential plant oils are rubbed into the skin to produce beneficial effects in the body.
Shiatsu an ancient Japanese massage system based on a knowledge of acupuncture points.
Reflexology a system of foot massage that has effects on other parts of the body.
Acupressure in which fingers—instead of needles— are used to stimulate acupuncture points.
Touch-for-health a system involving muscle testing.
Swedish massage probably the mother of all Western mainstream massage techniques.

Some of these forms of massage are considered in more detail in Chapter Five. They are not, however, the main concern of this book because we are not concentrating on therapeutic massage, meant to alleviate suffering or to cure medical ailments. This book looks at the other two areas of massage – sensual and erotic massage. These are primarily couple-centered methods of massage whose aim is the giving and receiving of pleasure rather than the curing of physical ills. Needless to say, by increasing emotional well-being, such methods do have beneficial effects on the individual's body and mind and thus could be said to be "curative" in the widest sense of the word. Certainly, it is my personal experience that couples who massage one another feel better not just in their relationship with one another but in their own general health and sense of well-being.

Why bother with sensual and erotic massage?

Over the years many couples have asked me why they should bother with sensual and erotic massage. After all, they argue, they have a good or reasonable sex life and communicate well enough on most things, so why give themselves yet another commitment to fit into their busy lives?

I think this argument highlights what is so wrong with many relationships today. And this is why, as a marital therapist, I place such importance on learning and using these techniques, and teach them to my patients.

Sensual and erotic massage is worth taking trouble over for the following reasons:

It encourages couples to create time and space in which to be alone together This is something that many do not otherwise bother to do. Most couples I see would benefit from spending much more time together, taking the trouble really to get to know one another. Many couples who do lots of things together and perhaps enjoy a social whirl that is the envy of others rarely spend time with one another alone, sharing and loving in the quietness of their relationship. Instead of simply being, they pour their energies into doing all the time. Far too many of us spend our lives doing rather than being. Needless to say, our relationships suffer as a result.

It costs nothing but time For even the least well-off couple, massage is something that they can share without financial cost. Most of us have come to think that we need to spend money in order to have fun. This is not so. The old truism that the best things in life are free was never more true than in regard to massage. It is also more readily and reliably available than sex.

It isn't goal-centered When couples come together for any kind of intimate activity it can end up becoming goal-centered. Men, especially, seem to have to set goals, however unconscious these may be, and women often find that this becomes tiresome or, eventually, even unacceptable. When you massage one another, however, it is enough simply to have as your goal that you please one another. There are no pressures to bring about an orgasm, and no failures due to fear. In short, the sole aim of giving or receiving a massage is pleasure for its own sake and this, unfortunately, is all too rare for most couples.

It is a fulfilling substitute for intercourse Many couples, as we have seen, see sex as being the only way that they can satisfy their need for touching. This is a shame, because touching and sex are not the same thing and yet massage can be as satisfying as either—and is wonderfully beneficial when, for any of the following reasons conventional sex is difficult or not possible.

- For most couples, at the time of the month when the woman is menstruating, vaginal sex is not acceptable.
- Pregnancy can be a time for sexual abstinence for others.
- A woman who has just had a baby or a gynecological operation will be sexually unavailable for a while.
- Anyone who is worried that he or she might have a sexually transmitted disease and especially anyone who fears that they or their partner are at risk of being HIV-positive is wise to avoid sex until they have been cleared by a doctor.
- Many thousands of women occasionally or regularly suffer from cystitis or thrush, or both, which makes it difficult or impossible to engage in sexual intercourse for a while. Herpes, too, rules out sex during an attack.
- Millions of people have sexual dysfunctions such as painful intercourse, or disorders of ejaculation or orgasm at some time in their lives.

And so on. Instead of such couples retreating from sexual activity entirely, as many do (if they do not seek solace outside their relationship, that is), they could use sensual and erotic massage as a highly pleasurable and rewarding alternative until their usual sexual activities can he resumed. It is a tragedy that I see daily—that far too many couples behave as though their sexual lives were over at the first sign of failure, illness, or disappointment. If only they knew how to touch one another in a loving and healing way in sensual and erotic massage, many an affair would be prevented and many a marriage enriched instead of being destroyed.

It is a valuable addition to intercourse Over many years together most couples find that, sexually, they become at least a little bored with one another. They probably made love for some time before settling down and then experienced the stresses and strains of young family life, with consequent restrictions on their privacy—and opportunities to be alone together. The sparkle is lost, the sexual champagne becomes flat and many begin to think of looking elsewhere. All my clinical experience has taught me that it is usually more worthwhile to invest effort in restoring the relationship you have than to start again, and sensual and erotic massage can be a great help in making this happen.

Many couples have told me how massaging one another started them off on a totally new road after many years of thinking that they knew everything there was to know about one another. This comes about partly because, when sensitively done, massage takes the receiver back to his or her earliest days of life as they abandon themselves to the wonderful sensations. In psychological jargon this is known as "regression" and it can have profound effects. Many say that massage puts them in touch with feelings they never knew they had; that it is a sort of mystical experience, a kind of meditation, and not just for the receiver but also for the giver.

This can mean that emotions start to be revived either at the time or afterwards, and these feelings can greatly deepen the relationship. Couples tell me that after a really loving massage session they feel closer than ever before. Indeed, it is almost impossible to feel hostile to someone who has just massaged you well and this is why couples who regularly massage one another rarely row. This basic, return-to-the-womb trust brings to most relationships enormous benefits that some people pay a fortune to achieve via professional therapy. Massage, then, can enhance a relationship that has begun to tarnish, and it does so in ways that cannot be foreseen or even believed by those who have no experience of them.

It makes sex better We shall look at this benefit in detail on page 60; suffice it to say here that most couples find that by taking the pressure off sexual performance they enhance their pleasure on the occasions when they do have sex. Many people, men in particular, use sex to achieve emotional ends that should not be reached by sex and many are delighted to be relieved of the need to perform. In effect, they are being given permission to enjoy nongenital closeness and intimacy.

It is the best way of improving communication
Few of us communicate as well as we could with our partner and sensual massage is a wonderful way of learning how to do so. We see on page 18 how this happens.

It is pleasantly relaxing Many of us relax very little in today's hustle and bustle but to do a massage properly entails making time and space, and relaxing together. For many couples sex itself is not very relaxing, colored as it is by all kinds of unconscious (and, of course, perfectly conscious) pressures such as:

- Fears of failure
- Having to perform
- Differences in sexual appetite
- Differences of sexual tastes and styles
- One partner not feeling like it when the other does
- Fears of pregnancy

These and a host of other hazards disturb the marital bed in most households, if only some of the time.

Sensual and erotic massage does away with all this and gives most couples a reliable way of pleasuring one another and relaxing into the bargain.

Setting the scene

You don't need much in order to be able to massage your partner. You will need to care enough to want to do it, of course. You will also need time; and a certain amount of energy and skill are vital. Also, there is a small amount of equipment that will help. But however you do it you will need to set the scene so that the experience is the best it can possibly be for both of you.

Creating the right environment

Creating the right environment is worth effort. Of course, you can carry out a massage out of doors if it is warm enough and you have the necessary privacy, and you can do a "quickie" massage almost anywhere that is comfortable but, for the best results, here are some tips that couples have found useful.

Take the phone off the hook Most of us are at the beck and call of our telephone and especially our cell phones whether at work or at home but there's nothing so guaranteed to wreck a relaxing massage as the insistent ring of the phone. So, if you have an answering machine, turn down all the settings and if you can actually unplug the phone or turn off your cell phone, do so!

If you are not alone in the house put up a "Do not disturb" notice This keeps children or other adults out, though most people tend to massage one another at night so that interruptions are not such a problem. This does, however, have another disadvantage, as both of you may be tired at the end of the day.

Dim the lights Massaging one another should be relaxing, so turn off harsh lights. You need just enough illumination so that you can see what you are doing. You could fit a dimmer switch to your normal lighting or candlelight is very soothing and romantic. Some people become very adept at doing it in the dark. Indeed, ancient Oriental masseurs were often selected from the blind because their sense of touch was already so enhanced by their having to rely on it.

Warm the room Ideally, the temperature should be about 75°F/24°C. The best form of heat is that provided indirectly by a radiator. Fan heaters are noisy and distracting and tend to create a draught of hot air over a small area. Switch on the heating at least half an hour before you intend to begin the massage session. Some people also find that they need to keep the receiver warm by putting a blanket or towel over the parts of the body not being massaged. Some couples use an electric blanket in the winter. However you achieve the right degree of warmth, ensure that you are warm whether you are giving or receiving massage. Either one or both of you can get tense muscles if you are too cold and this will hinder the massage process or even make it a waste of time.

Put on some music if this is what you like Some people find music very relaxing and others, a distraction. Do not use CDs that have lyrics—stick to music alone for best results.

Prepare a firm surface on which to massage your partner While it is tempting to use the bed it is best not to do so because so much of the energy you put into the massage ends up being dissipated into the mattress. It is far better to use the floor. Put a couple of folded blankets, a pad of foam, or a sleeping bag down and cover them with a sheet. The area covered by the padding should be large enough to accept not only the receiver's body but also your own knees. If you are uncomfortable you will not be able to give a good massage and your tension and discomfort will be transmitted to the receiver.

Raise the receiver's head with a thin pillow This makes the neck much more comfortable. Similarly, when the receiver is on his or her back place a small pillow under the lower legs or behind the knees; this will help the receiver's lower back to rest in a more comfortable position. As about half of the massage takes place with the receiver on his or her back, this reduces backache and makes the whole process much more relaxing.

Both giver and receiver should remove any jewelry
Watches, rings and body jewelry not only get in the way, they can cause pain or even damage in certain situations. It is best therefore to remove all such items to be on the safe side.

Undress to leave as few clothes as you feel comfortable with Ideally, you should both be naked—but if the room is not as warm as recommended the giver should wear light, unrestricting clothing.

Preparation Because massage involves skin contact, cleanliness is important. Some couples like to bathe or shower together first, perhaps starting to massage one another a little in the water as a pleasant preliminary. This can be highly enjoyable if you use a loofah, shampoo brush, or bath mitt to gently massage your partner.

If you have neither the time nor the opportunity to bathe with one another do at least ensure that your hands are clean if you are the giver. And keep your fingernails short so that you don't accidentally scratch your partner.

The hands are the main tools of the giver so take every care to keep them smooth and sensual. Keep your fingers flexible, too, if necessary by practicing some kind of close work that involves fine detail such as embroidery or modelmaking. This is especially likely to be useful if you normally do manual work and your hands have become used to coarse movements. Practice makes perfect in massage, as in most skills, so don't be disheartened if initially you find that you are not as dexterous as you or your partner would like. Follow his or her guidance and you will soon begin to get it right.

Don't forget that much of the effect you'll be having will come from the natural healing that we all have in our hands. The "laying on of hands" is an ancient practice recorded throughout history. Modern technology actually allows us to measure the healing forces and energy flowing through the hands as people concentrate on healing with them.

It is thought that the energy transfer that takes place during massage is the most vital part of the procedure.

Do not massage each other after a heavy meal or if you have had much to drink; both can spoil, or even totally ruin, a massage.

Silencing your mind is also an important part of the preparation for a good massage. Try to put any troubles of the day out of your mind and concentrate deeply on what you are about to do. An absent-minded or physically exhausted giver is a real menace to the receiver who will in turn receive very little. So, fill your mind with caring compassion for your partner.

Some precautions Massage is a natural healing method and a relaxing form of recreation yet it is not without dangers in certain situations. Never massage any areas where any of the following conditions are present:

- Fractures
- Open wounds
- Sores
- Boils
- Infectious rashes
- Easily damaged veins (especially in the legs)
- Bruises
- Lumps or tumors
- Inflamed joints
- Thrombosis or phlebitis in the legs
- Anyone who has a fever

Where necessary seek medical help to get these sorted out before proceeding.

Giving and receiving Although I refer throughout the book to the "giver" and the "receiver," in a sense this is misleading because massage is all about sharing. In one sense, the receiver is just as much a giver as the "giver." During a massage the two participants exchange energy flows and communicate intimately whatever their role in the massage session.

The receiver gives his or her trust and is totally vulnerable to the giver who, in turn, opens up all his or her channels of communication in order to be sensitive and aware of the needs of the receiver. In fact, being a receiver can be more difficult than being a giver because most of us find it more difficult to be totally relaxed, passive and vulnerable than to be "doing."

If you are the receiver, allow yourself to become totally passive. Shut off your awareness of the outside world; focus, perhaps, on a pleasurable scene and really live through it. Close your eyes and focus on your breathing or what is being done to you. Or even empty your mind totally. The only "duty" of the receiver is to let the giver know if certain parts of the massage are more—or less—enjoyable and to lovingly guide him or her as and when necessary. At first this will mean talking but after a while your partner will know what your needs are by your responses: the little moans, groans, sighs, subtle body movements, and so on that you make as the massage progresses.

If you are the giver your role is to be open to what your partner wants and best enjoys and then to fulfil his or her wishes. We shall now see how this can best be achieved.

Communicating through touch

Many of us think that the only way to communicate with our partner is to talk. But this isn't necessarily always the case. We communicate all the time, and often without talking. Nonverbal communication is probably responsible for more of what goes on between human beings than is talking. In spite of this many couples I see are rather bad at reading the cues from one another.

This is where sensual massage is useful. By really listening to your partner early on as you learn what he or she best likes you not only encourage openness but learn how to get it right for him or her. The only responsibility of the giver is to make the massage really pleasurable for the receiver, whatever this takes.

This usually means discarding all kinds of pre-conceived ideas as the receiver redefines what you thought he or she liked.

All of this give and take is extremely helpful in a couple's sexual life because most will come to behave in bed in the same way as they do on the massage mat. Remember, it is not enough to make assumptions on which you then structure your massage; you must be guided by your partner's expressed needs at the time. A willingness to be flexible and to throw out old notions of what "should" be pleasant will bring great benefit to your sexual life as you transfer similar communication skills and openness to the bedroom.

As time goes by you will be so good at "reading" your partner that talk will become unnecessary. You will be able to communicate at a much deeper level, reading quite subtle body language that before would have gone unheeded.

I believe that couples who massage one another also become more spiritually attuned. They start to communicate on a higher plane both when they are massaging one another and when they are not. This can only be to their advantage.

However, communicating at this level when massaging your partner does take practice, knowledge and skill. Here are some tips on how to give a massage.

Start off by lying down next to one another either flat on the floor or bed, or lying in the "spoons" position on your side with your front against your partner's back. Synchronize your breathing so that you breathe in and out at the same time. Relax and lose yourselves in this togetherness.

Remember that the sort of massage I am describing in this book is about relaxing and feeling safe. This feeling of trust must never be broken. This means always supporting the part being massaged. Even if your partner falls asleep, he or she should be able to feel totally confident that they are in good hands.

- If you are the giver, ask your partner if there are any particular parts of his or her body that feel in special need of attention.

- Balance your body so that your torso is mainly

upright and straight. Let your shoulders hang loose and be sure that you are not tense as you do the massage. Any tension comes across to the receiver and can ruin a massage.

• Focus your attention on your partner. Concentrate on your hands as you massage and always be open to what he or she wants.

• A good massage should feel like one continuous sequence, so take care you always have one hand in contact with the receiver's body to ensure this continuity.

• Keep the strokes reliably smooth and rhythmic. Work slowly and your partner will get the best out of the massage. There should be no surprises for the receiver—just a flow of predictably enjoyable strokes and movements.

All of these things will help to create the right mood and ensure that true communication takes place. Sensual and erotic massage have nothing in common with fixing the car and are largely intuitive processes of sharing, involving a total commitment to what you are doing and to the person with whom you are sharing the experience.

What you will need
Unless you want to invest in a proper massage table, and few couples do, the only things you will need are some oil or powder with which to lubricate the skin and perhaps a few pieces of special equipment to make the massage more enjoyable. Let us look at these in more detail.

Oils
Oils are used when massaging simply to make the contact between the skin and your hands more free from friction and thus more pleasant for the receiver as your hands glide over his or her skin.

The same effect can be obtained using talcum powder if you prefer not to oil the skin.

It is easy to overestimate how much oil is needed; a very small amount is sufficient to lubricate the skin. If you are too lavish, the oil will run over the contours of the body and onto the sheet underneath. Too much oil also reduces the amount of contact you can make, which is in itself a disadvantage.

Once you have oiled one part of the body (oil each part only when you are ready to massage it rather than all at once), that application should be sufficient for the whole massage, except when working on big areas such as the back, or very hairy zones—especially in men.

What sort of oil you use is up to you but do not feel that you must use fancy oils. You do not need to spend a fortune. Any vegetable oil, such as sunflower, safflower, or coconut is perfectly acceptable. Many beauty shops and chemists now sell inexpensive massage oils. You could even use olive oil but it is thicker and sticky. Mineral oils such as baby oil can also be used but they are not absorbed into the skin well.

Best of all, but most expensive, are aromatherapy oils. These are scented and can be tailor-made to have very specific effects—for example, they can be relaxing, invigorating, or erotic.

Various companies make plain massage oils that can be used as the base for your own personalized product. Simply add a few drops of your favorite perfume or aromatherapy oil.

Some people like to keep their oil in a dish but this can easily spill in use, so a flip-top bottle is best. This gives peace of mind while you are concentrating on the massage itself. Always warm the oil before starting, by putting the bottle into a bowl of hot water or by standing it a safe distance from a radiator.

When using the oil never put it onto your partner's skin direct from the bottle, because it can tickle unpleasantly or be cold. Always pour a little of the warmed oil into your hand first and then place that hand on your partner's body. Let it rest there for a moment and then slowly start to spread the oil over the area to be massaged. Make sure that your hands are relaxed and floating over the surface of your partner's skin. When making contact allow them to fall as if they were feathers. Similarly, when breaking contact with the skin do so gently and smoothly, never suddenly.

When you have finished the entire massage, your partner's body will be slightly oiled all over. Have a small towel handy to remove the excess.

Equipment

An electric vibrator is a useful tool for massage but be sure to use it before you start the massage proper. Although they have become associated with sexual arousal, vibrators can be useful for their original purpose! Even the phallic-shaped ones designed for clitoral stimulation can be good for short bursts of massaging. The best, though, are the electrically operated ones that can be attached to the back of your hand, so that it is your hand rather than the plastic or rubber of the gadget that makes contact with the body.

It is possible to buy numerous types of massage equipment and most of the large electrical companies have their own version. "Personal massagers" have different heads that can be interchanged for use on various parts of the body. While many women (and some men) use them for sexual arousal they also make fine massagers and if you have no partner or your partner is unavailable, you can use them to give yourself a massage.

A sauna or Jacuzzi can be a wonderful addition to your massage routine but most of us have neither the money nor the space for such luxuries. A really good bath is worth investing in though because if it is large enough you can bathe together as a lead-up to your massage. A power shower is within the reach of many families and this can be a good form of preliminary water massage before progressing to the real thing.

Various body rollers and similar devices are available from specialist health shops, pharmacies, spas, and the Internet, and they, too, are worth experimenting with.

For the vast majority of couples, however, massage can be wholly satisfying as a person-to-person affair in which they use only their hands.

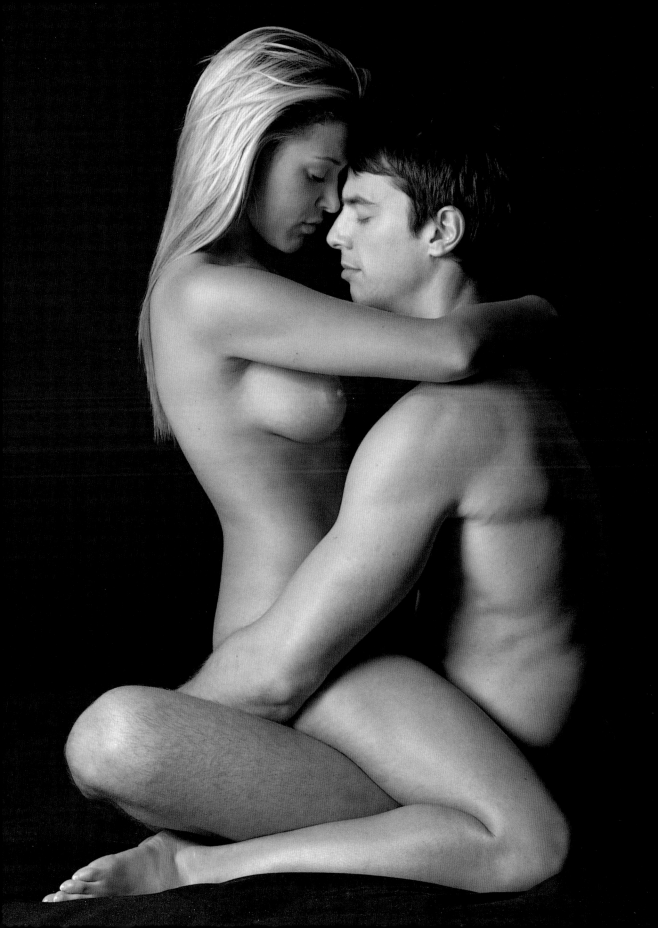

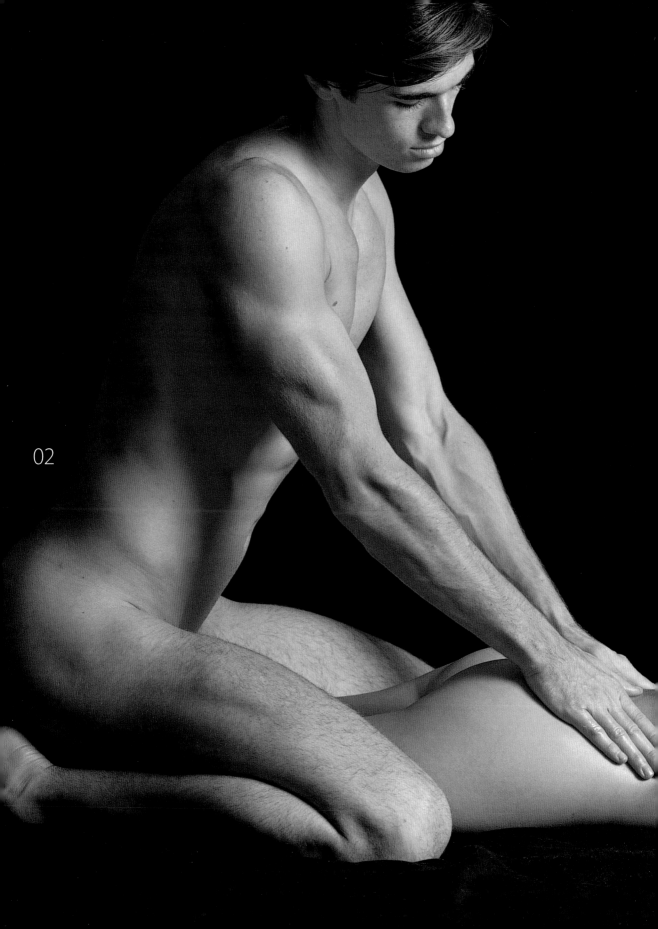

02

Some basic strokes and techniques

The main thing to remember when massaging your partner is that your intuitive feelings should be your guide rather than anything written here.

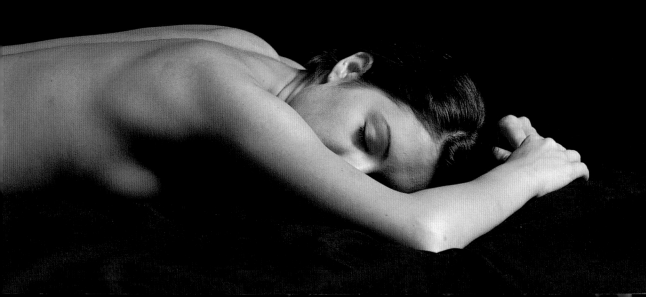

There is no right or wrong way to massage, do whatever feels good for the receiver and then patiently learn how to make it even better. Most couples gradually improvise their own methods—techniques that particularly suit them—and it is certainly not essential to become an "expert" at massage. However, it helps to learn certain basic skills so that you can both get the best out of the sessions you share together.

Many of my couples are delighted to learn some formal skills because this opens new doors for them. What at first may seem a chore to learn soon becomes natural and, like driving, becomes second nature once you are experienced. The actual manual skills then function automatically, leaving you free to enjoy the giving and receiving. So, if at first it seems like rather a lot to think about, don't panic—you will be surprised how quickly you improve, with practice.

There are literally thousands of ways of touching your partner but here let us first look at the techniques that are useful for sensual massage. (Erotic massage, discussed on pages 56–115, calls for rather different methods.)

It is useful to think of the basic sensual massage strokes and movements in three main groups: gliding, medium-deep, and deep. A fourth category—percussion—will also be described but I don't find that many couples use it much.

fingertips you can do a stroke called feathering—or butterfly strokes. This gives a lot of pleasure but requires some practice because early on it is easy inadvertently to tickle your partner and so spoil their relaxation.

Using the fingertips of both hands at the same time, or of each hand alternately, run them lightly over the skin. Travel down along the length of the body with these light brush strokes, perhaps overlapping your hands as you use first one and then the other. This is a useful stroke with which to end the massage session or to end work on any one part.

Long stroking movements are nice, too. In these you place your hands flat on your partner's body and then lean forward to slide them down (or up) the receiver's body as far as you can reach. Then circle your hands around and make the return journey. In this way you can cover large circuits of flat areas of the body, such as the chest, stomach, torso, or back.

Try making big circles with your hands one after the other, each overlapping the track of the previous hand so that they each form only part of the circumference of the circle.

Experiment with different speeds and pressures of all these strokes to see what your partner best enjoys. It is a good idea to practice on yourself first to get the hang of what different strokes feel like, and to get the pressure right.

Gliding
These strokes are some of the most sensual, and are easy to do. You simply let your hands glide gently and rhythmically over the surface of your partner's skin. Use these movements to start and to finish a massage session, by making them large and expansive rather than focused on a particular area.

Such movements are very smooth and soothing, and for this reason are used to apply oil at the start of work on any particular area. You can do them with the flat of your hand applied to the skin and with your fingers spread apart or close together. The feelings are quite different, depending on which method you choose. If you lift your palm off the skin and just use your

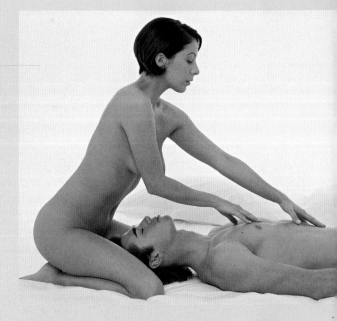

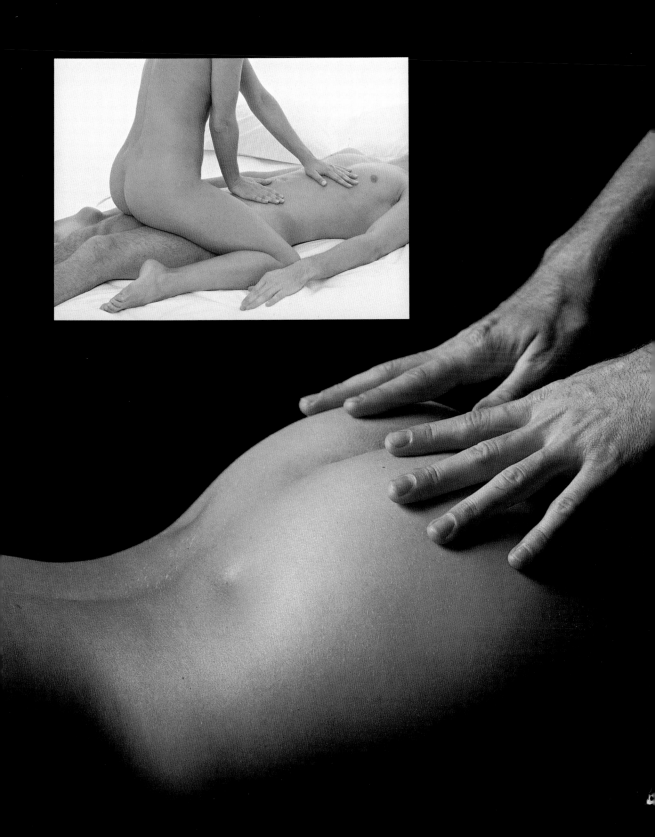

Medium-depth strokes

These use more pressure than gliding movements but do not go very deep into the muscles. A good one to start with is kneading. In this you take a "fistful" of flesh with one hand and squeeze it as if you were kneading dough. Then release it, at the same moment grasping a similar amount of flesh close by with your other hand, and so on. Make sure that one hand is always squeezing so that contact with your partner is uninterrupted.

Another stroke worth trying is a gentle wringing action, as if your partner's body were a large towel to be wrung out. Place your hands on either side of, say, the trunk and then bring your hands together quite firmly so that both come to lie in the center of the back. Now change hands so that the one that was pulling is now pushing, but from the other side of the body. This stroke works best on the torso but can also be used on the thighs.

A real favorite is a special form of pulling. Kneel at the side of your partner with your knees close to his or her body. Lean across and place both your hands on the opposite side of your partner's trunk, high up under the arm. Pull firmly on your right hand, drawing it toward the front of the chest and stopping just before you reach the nipple. Now do the same with your left hand, at the same time lifting off your right hand and returning it to the starting position but a little lower down the body. Continuing to use right and left hands alternately, gradually work your way down the body, overlapping the tracks you have just made until you reach the knee. Stop here and, returning to your starting point on the chest, begin the movements again.

Deep strokes

Harder to do and more tiring to perform, these call for some strength or the use of your body weight if you are slight. Because it is easy for these highly rewarding strokes to tire the giver, technique is more important here.

Never start off with these deep strokes. Always begin with gentle, soothing and relaxing movements. Once you have gained the confidence and trust of your partner you can progress to the deeper strokes. From my experience these are likely to call for much more feedback because you will be more likely to produce adverse sensations if you become too enthusiastic.

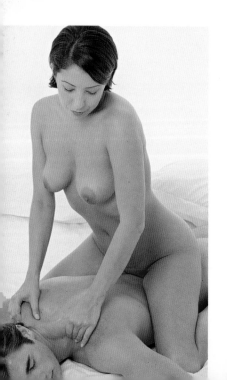
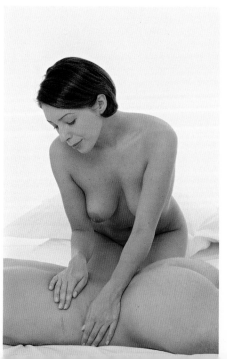
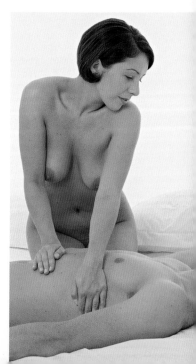

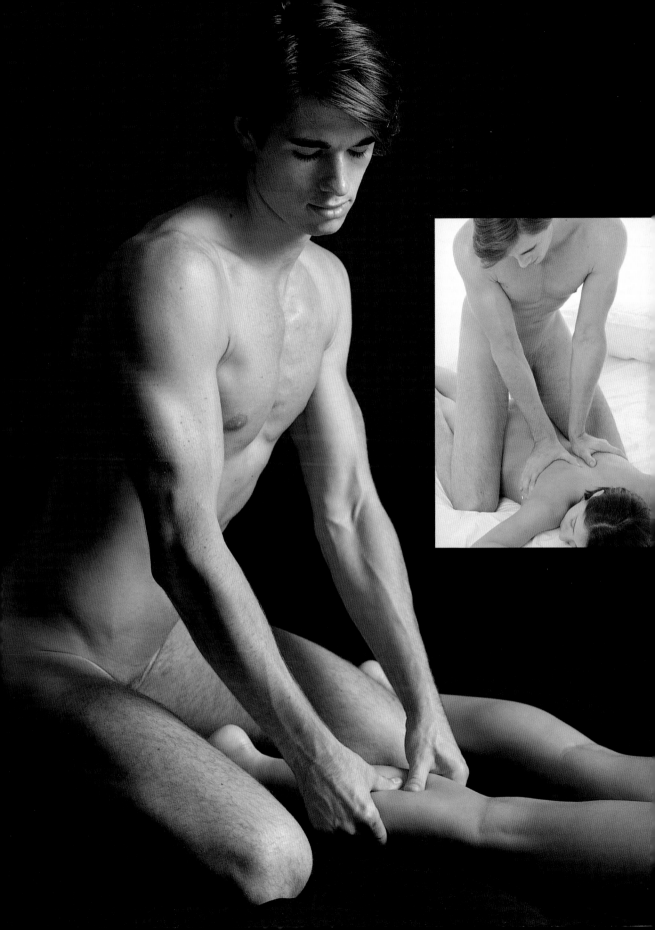

Having said this, many people are surprised by just how hardy the body is. Be guided in part by the amount of fat and muscle your partner has. Obviously a small, light person will be more easily hurt accidentally than one with a fair covering of fat and muscle, but common sense and some feedback during the first few sessions should quickly sort out such matters.

While talking about experiencing or inflicting pain during massage, there is sometimes a delicate balance between just enough firmness to make the stroke feel really good and going over the barrier into real pain. Again, experience will teach both of you just where this barrier is over your first few sessions together.

Perhaps the most popularly used of the deep strokes is that using the thumbs. Press the balls of your thumbs deep into the flesh, and using small circles, short strokes, or whatever you find best for each particular part of the body, push the skin away

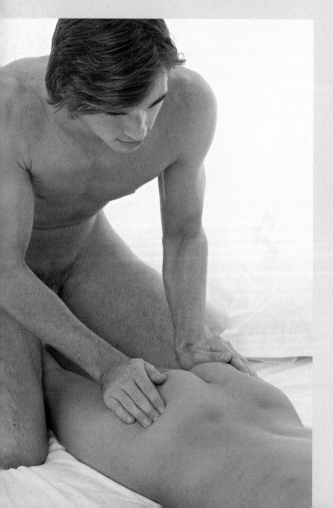

from you. Use the thumbs together or alternately and slowly work your way across the given area in a slow, creeping movement. Always keep one thumb in contact with the skin. A variant of this is to do the same massage but using the heel of your hand instead of your thumbs.

Fingertip pressure can be very effective, if tiring for the giver. Keep the tips of your fingers together, bunching them so that they form a multi-fingered pad of tissue. Push them deeply into the flesh and seek out any tense or painful areas that your partner tells you may need this form of relief. Get your body weight behind the movement and keep your arms straight or you will soon feel exhausted. It is possible, instead, to use just one finger, for specific well-defined points of tenderness or tension, but few people can keep this up for long.

Sensitive fingertip movements are good around joints, at the top of the back (around the shoulder blade), in the palm of the hand, and on the sole of the foot. Try them out on other areas.

Percussion This is less popular with couples doing sensual massage than with true masseurs, because this form of massage is stimulating rather than relaxing. However, it can be helpful.

Hacking is a form of percussion in which the sides of the hands alternately hit the receiver's body in a rhythmical way, all the time moving around the area being massaged. This works well on the buttocks, the thighs and the calves but can be painful elsewhere.

Pummeling is really hitting your partner with a loosely clenched fist. Again, it should only be done in areas where there is plenty of flesh. Never do it near or over bony areas, such as the ribcage or the front of the leg.

Pinching can be surprisingly pleasurable, too. Pinch small lumps of flesh with the fingertips of each hand in turn.

Sometimes these more invigorating techniques are useful as you proceed from sensual massage to erotic massage, if that is what you intend to do at any one session. They can easily lead on to foreplay.

If you master all of these strokes over just a few

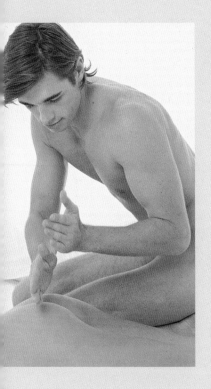
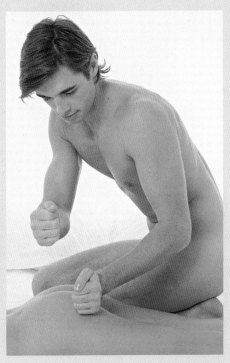
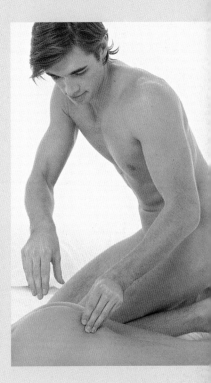

sessions and quickly come to know what your partner best likes, you will have done extremely well. It can take months to become an expert at recognizing your partner's needs and, of course, these will change from time to time. Women, especially, have differing needs according to the time of the month. This is particularly true of women who retain a lot of fluid in their tissues during the menstrual cycle. A manoeuvre that was highly exciting and enjoyable earlier in the month can become painful in the week before a period. Learning about such considerations makes a man more sensitive to his partner's body and its cyclical changes, and this greatly helps their sex life in general.

Having learned and mastered your basic strokes, keep on practicing and developing your own variations. Those I have described work well for most people but there is considerable scope for individual variation. This is a point worth making again and again because I find that some people, when massaging their partner, often concentrate on the areas and stroke types that they themselves best enjoy. Some find it difficult to believe that their partner enjoys something different and may even get quite annoyed because they cannot force their preference onto their

partner. This usually tells me a lot about the marriage and, indeed, the couple also learn greatly from talking it through.

You, too, can learn from how you communicate during a massage. Use the experience to see how well you actually listen to one another's requests and needs. How do you respond? How do you feel when you are asked to do something, especially if it is not what you think you should do or would prefer to do? Are you tense or anxious at having to receive? Do you find yourself always offering to give and rarely receiving? All of these, and many more, are useful areas for discussion within a loving relationship.

Many people of both sexes actually censor pleasure. It is as if they have been brought up to believe that it is wrong to feel good—and indeed many of them have. Such a person will need a lot of patient understanding from their partner to help them break free from such ingrained inhibitions and to allow their feelings of pleasure to come through. Try to be positive in your reaction to any such issues that arise as a result of massaging one another and seek professional help if things get too difficult for the two of you to handle alone.

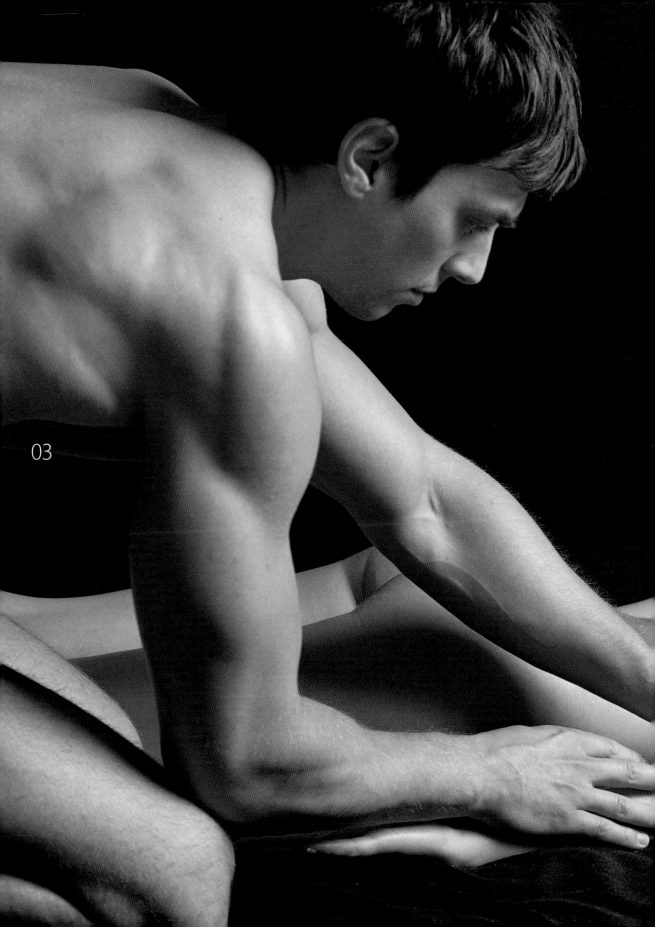

03

How to do a basic sensual massage

There is no absolute right or wrong way of doing a sensual massage, as I have said before, but however you decide to do it you will need to be systematic about it if you do not want to miss out on whole areas of pleasure for your partner.

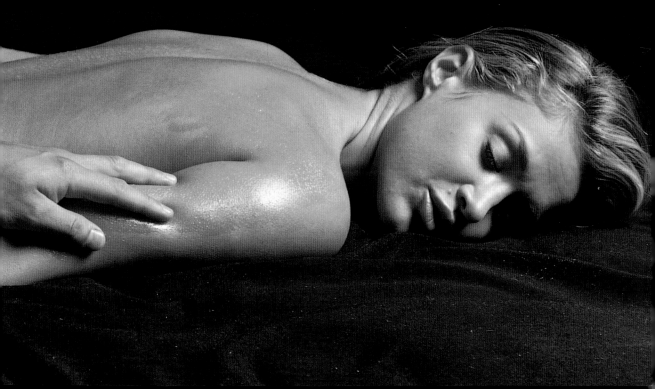

Having said this, it also depends on how much time you have at your disposal. Many massage books—and there are some good ones around—are written with the assumption that the couple has an hour or two to spend. If this is so you could work through the whole of the sequence described below; it takes about an hour to do thoroughly. However, if you have only half that time or even less, it does not mean that you have to put off giving and receiving until another day. Ask your partner what he or she would like best and then do a shortened version of the massage routine. A loving couple should feel free to ask for, and receive, what they want, whether this happens to be a back massage, ten minutes devoted to their feet, or whatever. It most certainly does not have to be "the whole production" or nothing.

Some of the things described below will be especially pleasant for certain individuals and yet for others may be positively unpleasant. Over the first few weeks of trying things out you will soon discover what you both like. The routine I describe below is somewhat full and I know very few couples who do it all every time. Nor should they, necessarily.

Giving and receiving a good massage has nothing in common with, say, following a cooking recipe. You do not have to follow a plan slavishly in order to be successful. In fact it is far better if you don't stick rigidly to a set routine. Early on, though, as when learning most things, it pays to be systematic and structured about it all. Later you will be able to take matters into your own hands and devise tailor-made sequences for your partner.

There is, however, one rule worth following: Do not touch the breasts or genitals in the course of a massage. A sensual massage is not aimed at sexual arousal—in fact arousal can detract from the pleasure. If, once you have completed your sensual massage, you want to go on to erotic massage or foreplay then, of course, the breasts and genitals will become centers of attention.

From my experience, the best place to start a massage is the back. So let's look at this first.

The back I suggest to couples that they start with back massage for many reasons.

- It is a relatively strong, flat part of the body, which makes it a good starting point while the giver gets into the mood and the receiver starts to relax and trust the giver.
- It is large and responds to many different types of strokes, thus allowing the giver to introduce variety into his or her repertoire—and produce good feelings for the receiver right from the start.
- Many people are very tense at the top of their neck and shoulders and doing something about this is a good start to a more generalized body massage.
- Back massage often makes the receiver so relaxed that he or she is then ready for the rest of the procedure to follow.
- Lastly—and perhaps as a therapist I see more of this than others do—if the individual being massaged lies face down at the beginning of a massage, he or she feels less vulnerable than lying face-up, particularly if naked.

All of these reasons make the back a good place to start.

First, the giver should get into a good, relaxed position. Because the back is so large, especially if the receiver is both tall and well built, you will be moving about quite a bit when doing long strokes. This can best be achieved by kneeling at the head of the receiver, who is lying facedown, flat on the floor, arms lying along his or her sides and the hands/palms upward. The head should be turned to one side. Your knees are either side of the receiver's head in this position.

Another favorite of mine is for the giver to "sit" astride the receiver's buttocks but taking care not to put any weight onto the receiver's body. This improves the sensuality of the massage because the giver's body is so intimately in contact with that of the receiver.

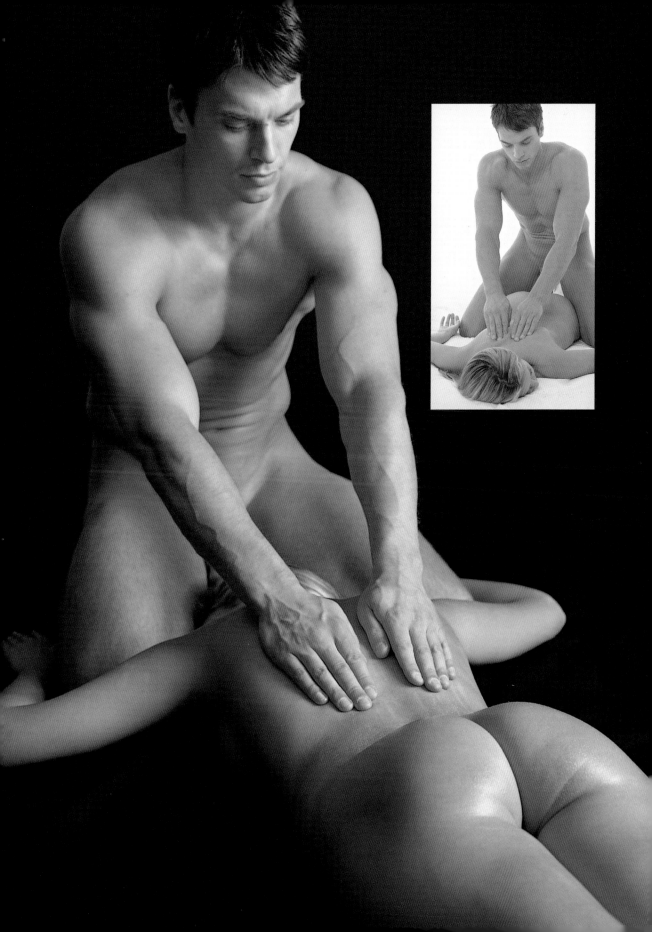

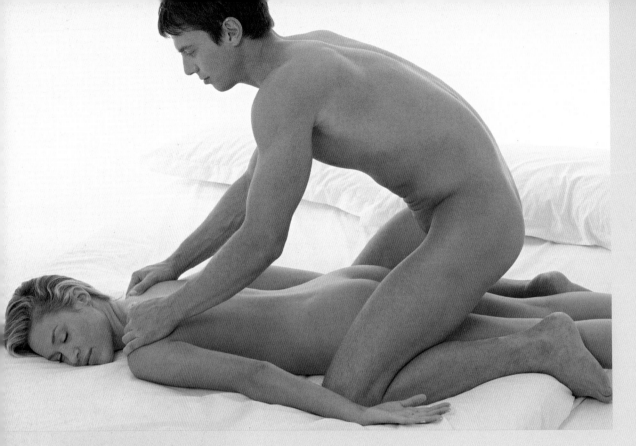

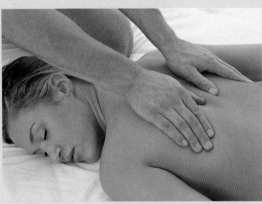

Now you are ready to start the actual massage. First, take a few slow, deep breaths in and out, at the same time relaxing your shoulders. Close your eyes if this helps and center your thoughts on your partner.

Then open your eyes and, taking a little warmed oil in the palm of one hand, lightly spread it all over your partner's back. Then close your eyes once more while you concentrate on the feel of the body beneath your hands. Do some long strokes up and down the back making large circles with both hands, each making the same movements but in a mirror image of one another.

Now, opening your eyes again, you are ready to work more firmly, using whatever strokes you find best, on the base of the neck, then the shoulders. Do one shoulder at a time and use kneading, thumb pressure and broad strokes thoroughly to massage the top of the back, seeking out any knotted or "gritty-feeling" areas. Work all around the shoulder blades, perhaps with the tips of your fingers, and then lift the shoulder with one hand while you continue the massage of this area. For this last part you will find it best to alter your position so that you are beside the receiver's chest and facing his or her head.

Now straddle your partner as before and, using your fingertips bunched together to form a pad, run them up and down the sides of the spine along the large muscles there.

Run your hands right from the base of the spine to the top of the back and then down again. Be guided by what feels good to your partner. Concentrate on such areas with deep, deliberate strokes. Then gently "walk" your fingers up and down the spinal muscles; take great care to avoid pressure on the spines of the vertebrae in the midline because this can be very uncomfortable.

End with some broad, integrating strokes that "smooth over" the whole back area.

So that you can massage the lower back with ease, reposition your body so that your knees are level with the receiver's thighs. Do some medium-deep circular movements with the hands overlapping their tracks around the base of the receiver's back. Go on to knead the buttocks, perhaps with the addition of some chopping movements, if the receiver likes this. With you at the receiver's side, leaning across to his or her opposite side, pulling up the sides of the buttocks can be good, too.

Make your hands broad and using big, circular motions, massage all over the buttocks from the lower back to the top of the thighs.

Now use your bunched fingertips again to probe deeply into the muscles of the buttocks, over the hip joint. Make small circles here until you find what is most pleasurable for your partner; such sensations here can come as a great surprise at first.

Now you should be ready to start on the legs.

The backs of the legs The best position in which to massage the legs is to open your partner's legs so that there is enough room for you to kneel between his or her feet and facing the body. Start by oiling both legs at once. This might mean leaning forward if your partner is tall. When both legs are oiled from buttocks to ankles, concentrate on one leg at a time.

The backs of the legs give very variable pleasure to different people. Some like their calves massaged yet get little or no sensation on the back of the thighs, and for a few it is the other way around. Whatever you do and however you do it, always bear in mind that it is best to apply very little pressure on the skin of the legs as you go down them. This is because it is easy to force blood into the valves that are arranged all along the veins in the legs and this causes pain or discomfort. It can also be dangerous if the individual being

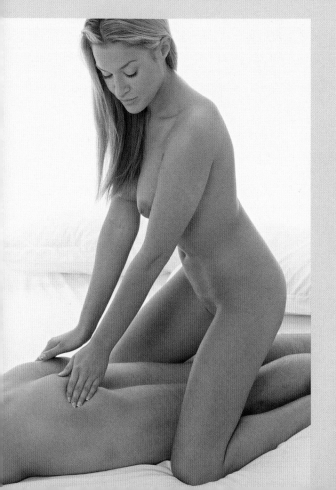
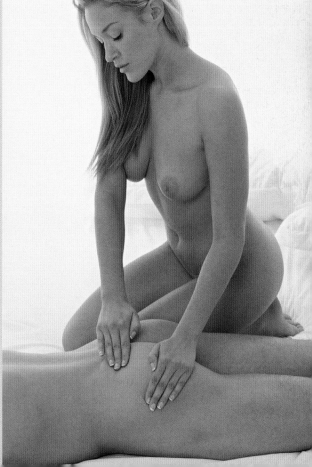

massaged has varicose veins, so, if there are varicose veins (these are fat, knotted, tortuous and easily visible) keep your massage well clear of them.

Kneading and wringing (see page 26) are good on the legs and two that I find go down well are the following:

With your partner still in the first position, raise his or her lower leg to a right angle with the floor. Sit forward and rest the sole of the receiver's foot flat against your chest, then massage the calf deeply, using both thumbs. Work up the calf firmly and repeat the movement in waves with both thumbs at the same level on the leg. Many people find this exquisitely sensuous.

Another favorite is to massage the insides of your partner's thighs. Sit comfortably astride his or her legs, level with the knees. Now massage deeply along the inner surfaces of the thighs up to, but not including, the genitals. This massage is usually very relaxing, especially for women.

Lastly, do some big, broad strokes from ankle to buttocks, running your hands over the buttocks and around the hips in large, circular movements.

Some people like to go on to the feet at this point but I find that it is easier to massage the feet when the receiver is on his or her back.

Before your partner turns over, do some gentle, preliminary work on the arms.

The backs of the arms Kneel at the side of your partner and do some long, flat-handed strokes down the arm on that side. Start at the shoulder and caress the arm with both hands alternately in a wave-like motion as they progress down the arm. Carry the stroke right down to the fingers and end the stroke at the fingertips very sensitively. Try to envelop the whole arm with these long strokes . . . the effect is wonderful.

Lastly, kneel between your partner's legs again, or sit over the backs of his or her knees, now close together, and do some long integrating strokes all over the back of the body from neck to knees. You can also go down the arms again if you like and can reach. This unites all the areas you have been massaging and ends this phase.

Some people stop here if this is all they have time for or if there is insufficient time for the giver to become the receiver as would be the case if the whole sequence in this chapter were to be done in its entirety. Let us assume, however, that you are continuing as the giver and your partner as the receiver. The next step is to ask him or her to turn over.

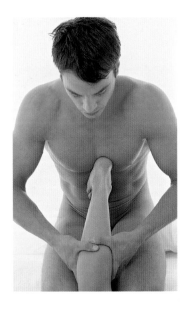
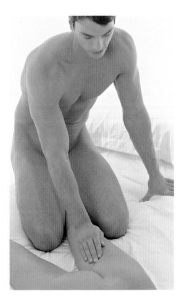
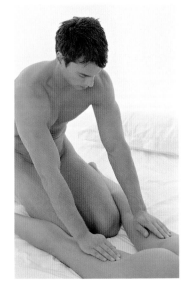

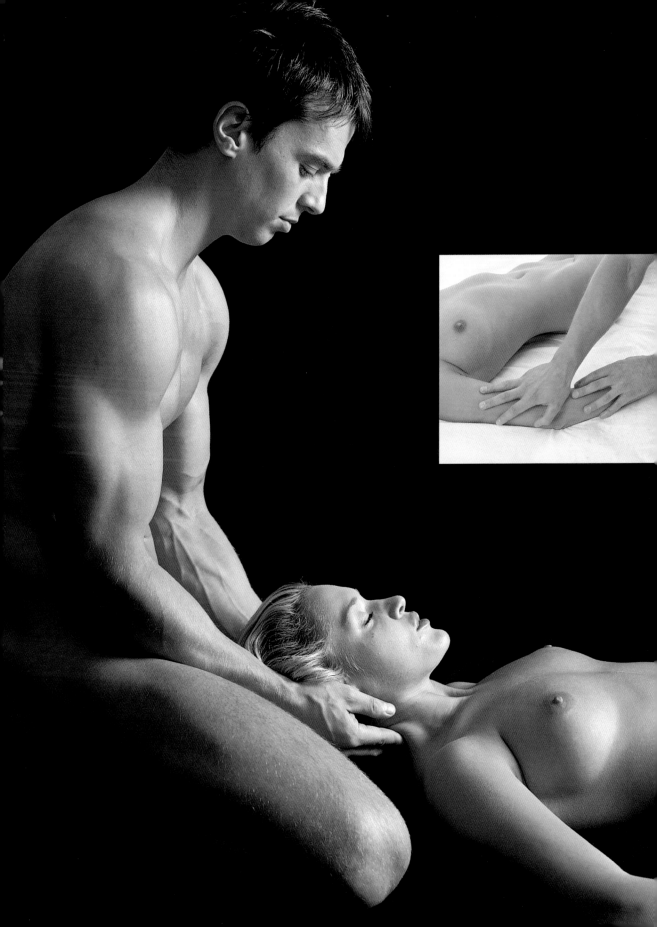

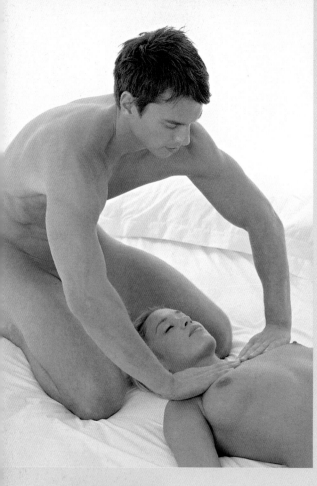

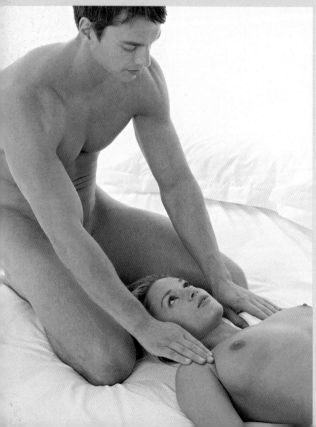

The shoulders and neck Once your partner is lying face up it makes sense to go back to the neck and shoulders because they are often still tense, even if your previous efforts were beneficial. Working on the shoulders and neck from the front (as in the large picture on page 37) can actually be more effective because the receiver's own weight assists your efforts. Kneel at your partner's head for this part of the massage.

Start, as always, by lightly oiling the area. With a little warmed oil on the palms of both your hands, begin by placing them on your partner's chest at the very top of the breasts. Let them rest there for a while with the fingertips of both your hands nearly touching one another over the breastbone. Now move the heels of your hands outward toward the shoulders and then around the back of them to the top of the shoulder blades. Now run them up the back of the neck. Repeat this stroke several times, starting at the top of the chest each time.

Next, take hold of your partner's head with your fingers at the base of his or her skull and gently pull the neck so as to stretch it. There is no danger in this, provided you do it gently. An extension of this is gently to stretch the neck forwards by inclining it slightly toward the feet, all the time stretching the neck. Then carefully lower the head onto the floor again and place your hands under the neck. Massage the back of the neck with one hand on one side and then, reversing the process, massage the other side of the neck with your other hand.

Lastly, massage the top of the back, above the shoulder blades and out to the tip of the shoulder but this time from underneath. You did something similar earlier, when your partner was lying on his or her stomach, but this way round is particularly pleasant to do and their body weight pressing on to your hands helps greatly.

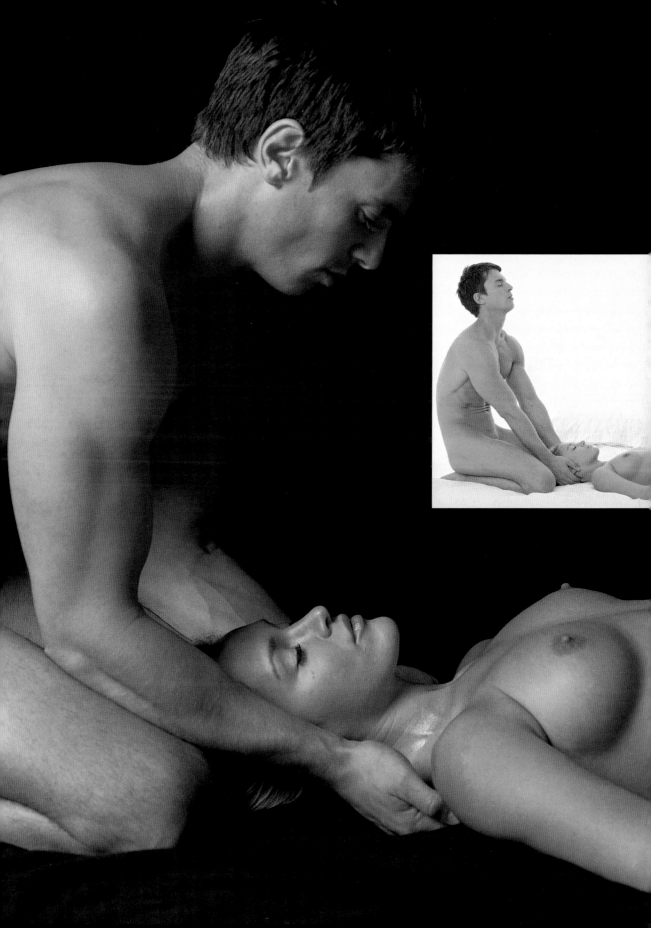

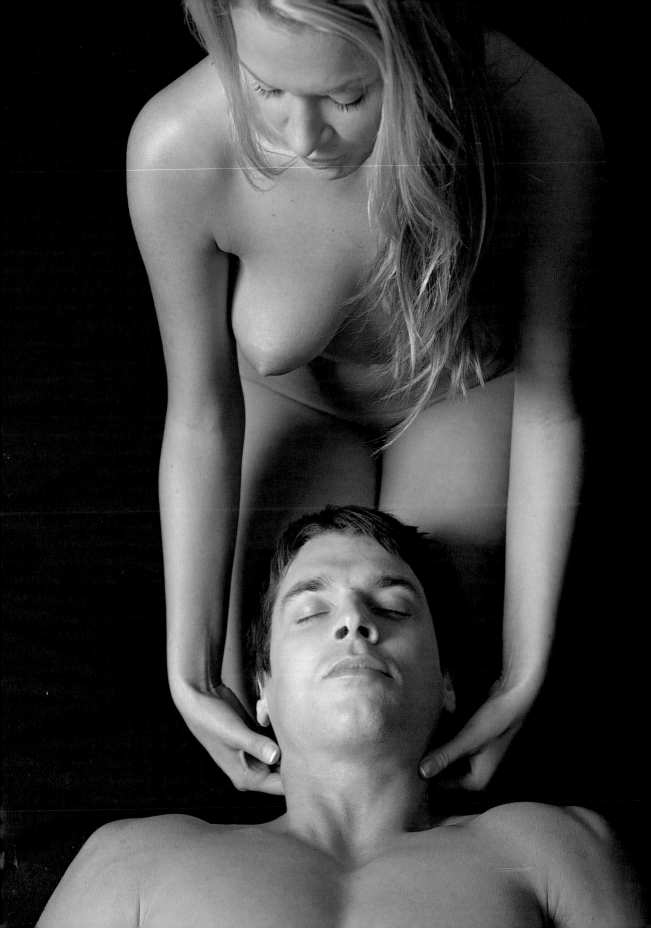

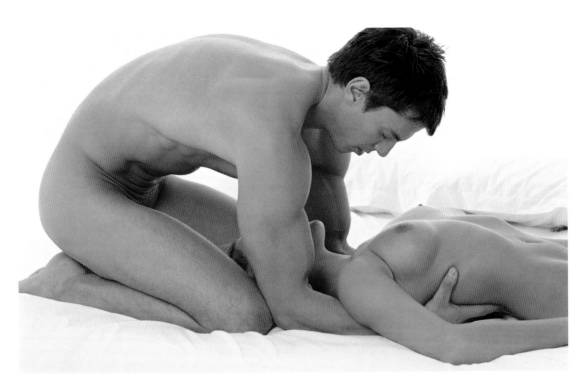

Spinal stretch Unless your partner is very heavy or large (in which case you will find it difficult or impossible to do) this is a very enjoyable maneuver for the receiver.

He or she should raise their head and back a little, so that you can get your hands and arms underneath. You then lean forward so that your body is virtually parallel with your partner's and reach right down to put your hands under his or her back and sides, level with the navel.

Now tell your partner to relax totally and go floppy on you. Keeping your hands still where they are, pull back with your body weight. This pulls on the lower half of your partner's body, which is fixed by its own weight. This feels lovely for the receiver.

Now let the surface friction between your skin and your partner's slip a little and allow your hands to glide up the back of his or her spine, along the big muscles at either side of the vertebrae. Allow your hands to travel right up the receiver's back as far as the shoulders, then on to the neck and lastly right up to the scalp. This produces a very unusual sensation which most people greatly enjoy.

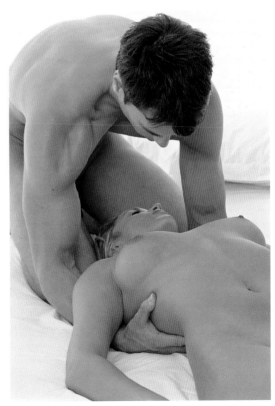

The face

Our face often reveals more of how we feel than does any other part of our body. Certainly, it is possible to read a lot from people's faces, both of their present and their past.

Massaging the face is an intuitive matter that calls for some experimentation to determine what feels good. You will not need to oil your hands again, because the small amount of oil you need will already be on them, from the massage you have already carried out.

Sit or kneel with your partner's head between your knees and gently explore what feels nice for him or her. The face is fairly bony, but don't worry about doing any damage; it is nothing like as vulnerable as it may look except for the fine skin around the eyes—be careful here. You could perhaps first try massaging your own face to get the hang of how it feels.

People experience very different sensations when their face is being massaged so it pays to listen carefully to the feedback from your partner while you are still learning.

Movements have to be small and controlled compared with those made on large areas of the body.

Make your movements slow, too, and very soothing.

Although massaging the face satisfactorily calls for quite a lot of experience if it is to be massaged according to your partner's wishes, here are a few movements that many people find pleasant.

First place your fingertips at the sides of your partner's head (near the temples) and your thumbs centrally on his or her forehead, at the hairline. Slide your thumbs apart slowly, toward the sides of the forehead, then return them to the center, but moving down a little, and repeat the process. Then, keeping your hands in much the same position, work on your partner's eyebrows in the same way.

Next, starting under the inner corners of the eyes work your thumbs outward over the cheeks to the jawbone. Move down the cheeks as you repeat this until the whole of the lower face has been covered.

Bunch your fingertips together and massage the chewing muscles up to the jaw joint, in front of the ear. Then massage the chin with gentle pinching movements.

Using the flat of your hands, massage the face all over, holding it in positions that are pleasant for your partner.

Finally, simply hold your hands over the receiver's face as a soothing end to the massage of this area.

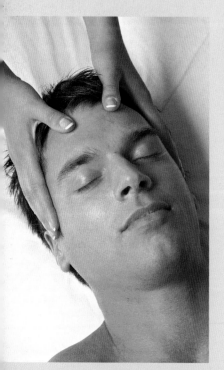
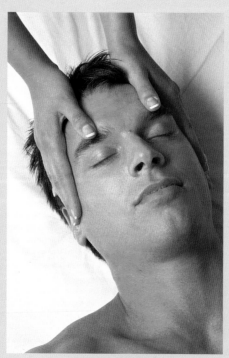
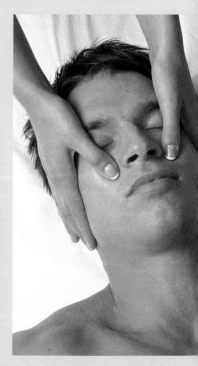

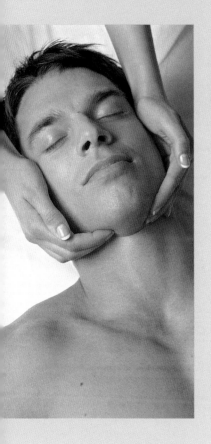

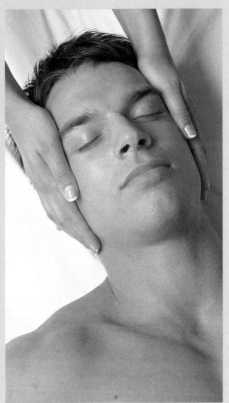

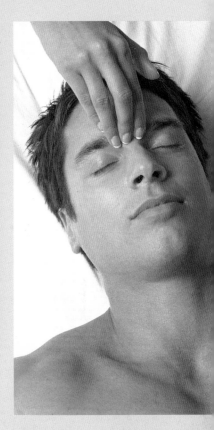

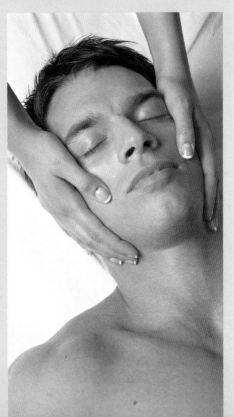

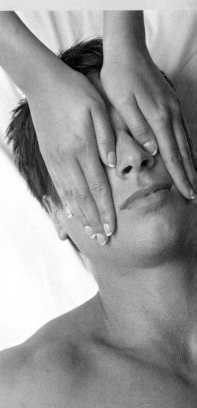

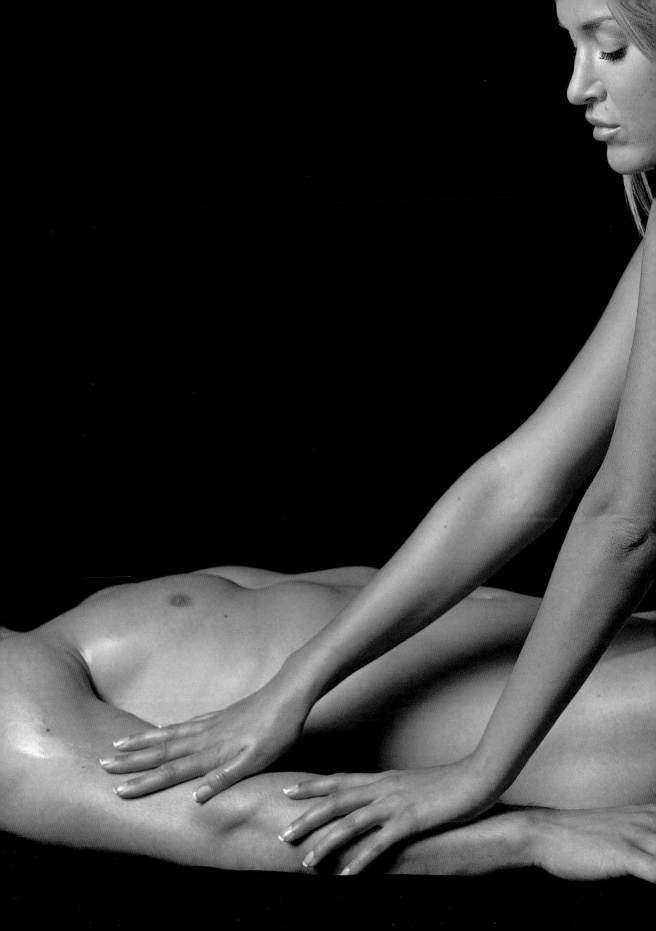

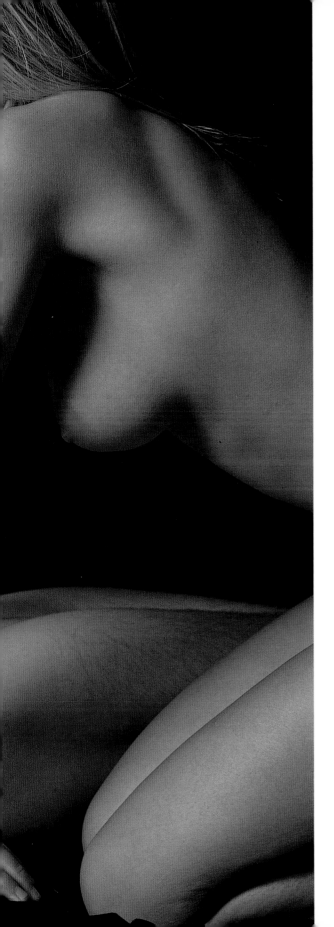

The arms and hands Massaging the arms and hands can be a valuable experience for those who tend to bottle up their emotions. They may find themselves clenching their fists, fiddling with things, drumming their fingers, or even wanting to hit out at someone they feel angry with. All of these emotions remain "tied up" in the arms and hands and great benefit will be derived from the release of these tensions.

Kneel beside your partner and lightly oil the arm from shoulder to hand, using your hands alternately in long, flowing strokes that overlap and work slowly down from shoulder to hand as you do this.

Just as I described for raising the foot and bending the knee on page 36, this technique is very relaxing for the receiver if you do the same with the arm. Raise your partner's forearm so that it rests on the elbow and hold his or her hand in one of yours. Enclose the wrist in your other hand and slowly but firmly move your hand down the forearm, squeezing it all the time as if you were milking fluid out of it. Repeat this several times as in the picture below.

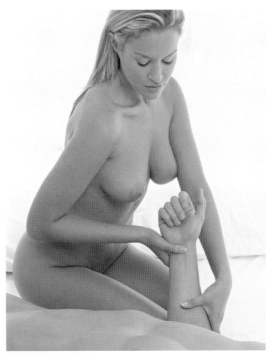

Next you can either knead or wring the upper arm. End with some long, integrating strokes of the whole arm and shoulder. Then repeat the whole process with the other arm.

The hand, too, is a remarkably enjoyable part of the body to have massaged yet it almost always comes as a surprise to people just how good it feels.

Start by asking your partner to rest his or her hand, palm up, on the floor then massage the palm gently. Then lift it up and, while holding it in one of your hands, use the thumb of your other hand to massage all over your partner's palm, asking as you do so where it feels best. Keep on exploring the palm until you have discovered all of the pleasurable areas and how he or she best likes them to be massaged. This can take some time. Indeed, like the feet (see page 52),

some people enjoy having their hands massaged for many minutes.

Now gently pull the fingers one at a time; be careful about this because the sensation can be a little alarming at first. Go gently so as not to cause tension or pain. Work first on one hand and then on the other while holding the hand at the wrist firmly and securely.

Next, place your palm against that of your partner's so that your fingers match up. Now slide your fingers between his or hers and bring them upward to your partner's fingertips. This delicious massage strokes the sides of the fingers and many people enjoy having this done for some time. Indeed, I have found that some people cannot get enough of these hand movements, so pleasurable are they.

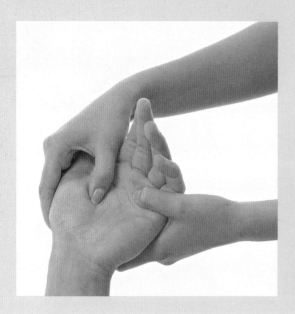

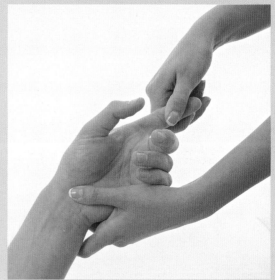

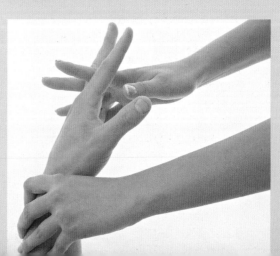

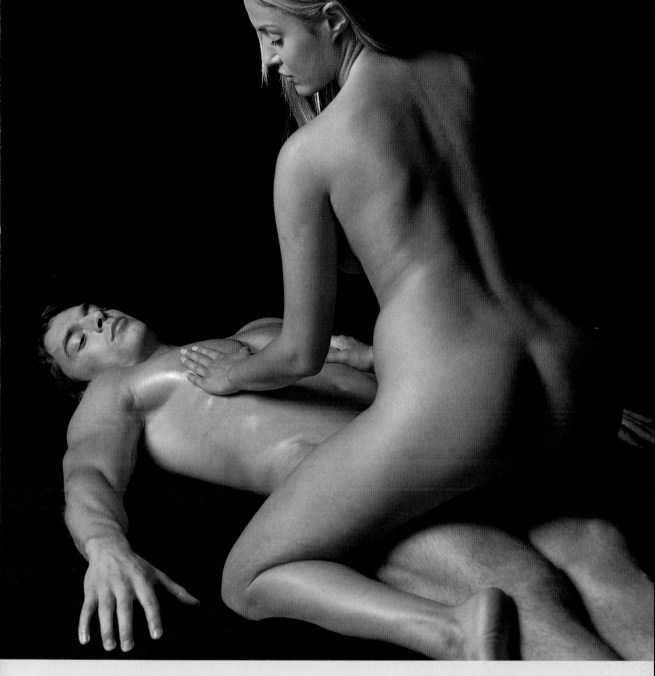

The chest and stomach There are
two positions that you can adopt when
massaging this area of the body. Some
people like to kneel by their partner's head
but I recommend kneeling astride the
receiver's closed-together legs. The skin-
to-skin contact of the giver's naked flesh
against that of the receiver then adds to
the intimacy.

Start by lightly oiling the whole area with long strokes,
then do some broad, circling motions over the chest,
using the flat of your hands. Don't forget that you
should avoid touching a woman's breasts during
sensual massage, so concentrate only on the top of
the chest if you are massaging a woman. Some
women find that the area just below the collar bone
gets quite tense and is pleasurable to have massaged.

Now (and for this you are best at your partner's
head) run your bunched fingertips along the grooves
between your partner's ribs. This should be modified

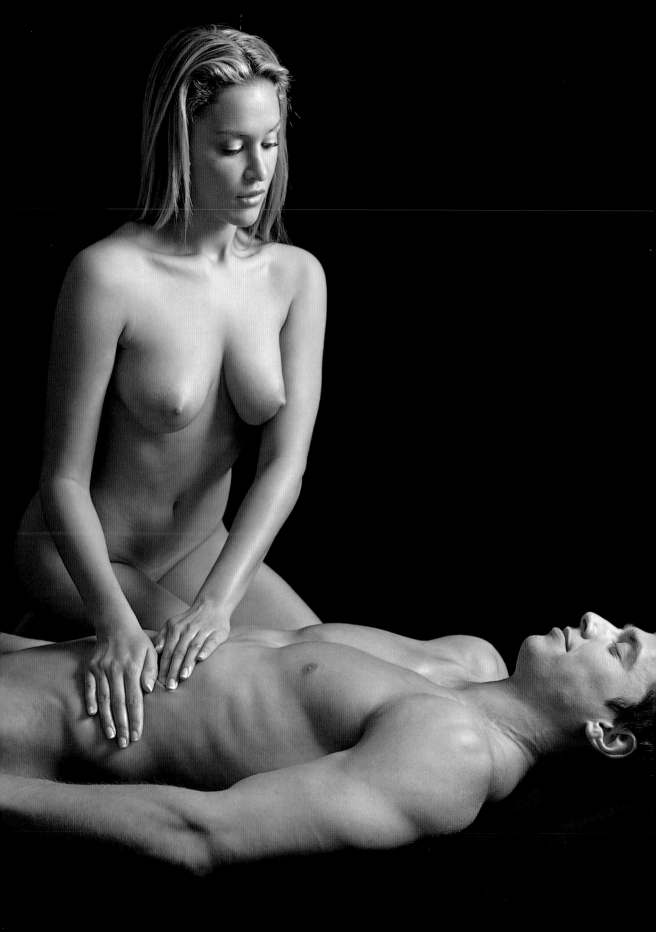

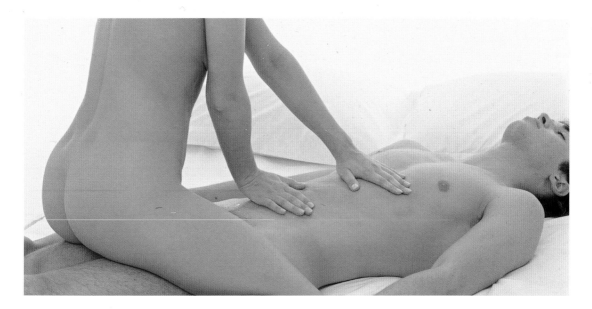

when massaging a woman because you will have to stop at the soft tissue of the breast and continue at the outer edge where it becomes ribcage again. You will become quite adept at this with practice. Above and below the breast area, the massage is the same as for a man.

Kneel on one side of the receiver with his or her arm on the opposite side stretched out at right angles to the body. Now, with plenty of oil on your hands, reach over and, working with pulling movements (see page 26), bring your hands upward from where the body meets the floor right up and over toward you, as far as the midline of the body. Do this using your hands alternately in a motion that takes them slightly farther down along the body at each stroke and pull with each hand slightly overlapping the track of the previous one. Carry on in this way until you reach the knee. Repeat the whole process from armpit to knee several times. Then kneel on the opposite side of the receiver and repeat the process again several times, massaging the second side. The idea is to make it seem as if there were one continuous wave of touch going down the whole length of the receiver's side.

I find that many people do not like to have their stomach massaged. Obviously, anything that tickles is counterproductive but this can be avoided if the giver keeps the strokes firm and purposeful.

Two forms of massage are pleasant for many people. The first is broad circling, using both hands at once and overlapping them as they pass each other. Start with one hand, palm down, just below the breastbone and the other just above the pubic hair. Move each hand round in a circle. The lower hand should move in complete circles while the other breaks contact as it crosses the first. From most people's experience the motion of both hands should be clockwise rather than counterclockwise. This is because food residues in the colon, just below the skin and muscle, are forced along it by the contraction of its muscular walls in a clockwise direction. This seems to be the way that energy flows in the skin and muscle of the abdomen. In fact, without explaining this I have, in the past, experimented with counter-clockwise movements—only to have the receiver ask me to stop at once because it felt so unpleasant.

Another motion that I find people enjoy on the stomach is small, circular movements, again going around within a larger circle. Imagine one of those whirling rides at a fairground in which each car rotates while the platform itself also spins around at speed. Mimic this at slow speed and you will be able to induce some lovely sensations in your partner.

Finish by doing some integrating movements to unite the whole of the chest and abdomen before going on to massage the fronts of the legs.

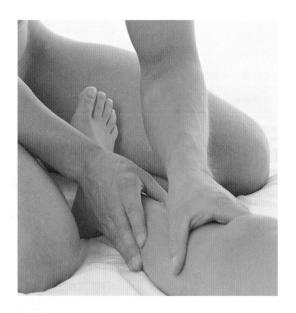

The fronts of the legs
This area is treated much like the back of the legs but with more caution when massaging the lower leg because the shinbone is so near the surface that pressure here can cause pain.

The best position for massaging this area is with you kneeling so that one of your partner's lower legs is between your knees. You could start off by kneeling between the feet, with the receiver's legs apart so that you can oil both legs. But as you work on one leg at a time you will eventually need to alter your position so that the leg being worked on lies between your knees.

Start with some long strokes from groin to ankle, each stroke covering a large area of skin with a broad hand movement. Either use both hands, with your fingers pointing up the leg and being drawn downward in waves alternately, or cup your hands across your partner's thigh or lower leg and move them alternately downwards in an overlapping pattern. Retrace this path but now with your hands more to the side of the leg. Then repeat it on the other side. In this way you will cover the whole leg in about three journeys.

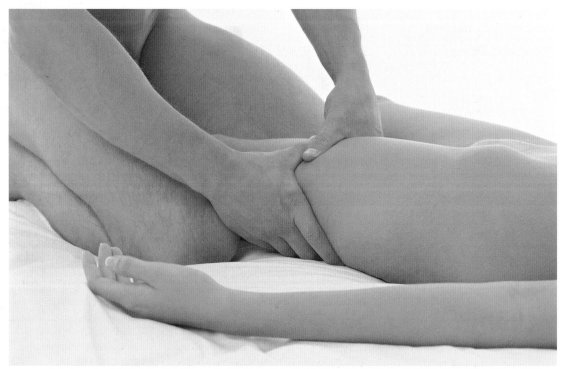

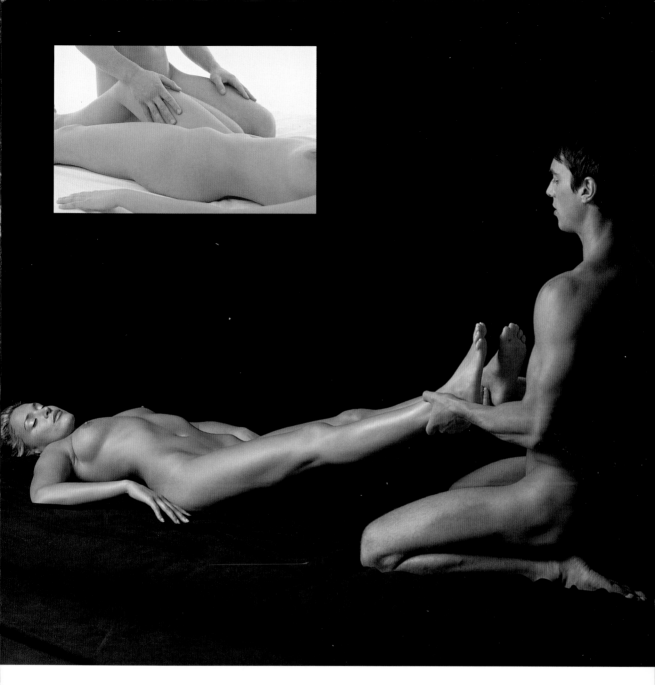

This can be repeated depending on what you have time for, and according to your partner's desires.

The thigh can be pleasantly massaged in two more ways. First, using your thumbs, work up from the knee to the groin, perhaps with the leg bent at the hip and the knee. See what feels best for you and your partner. "Milk" the tissue, using your thumbs together, pushing in the same direction and gradually working up the thigh inch by inch until you reach the groin.

Secondly, massage the inside of the thigh and especially the "tunnel" between the muscles from knee to groin. Some people like this to end with a massage of the groin area where the leg joins the stomach.

Lastly, kneeling at the feet of your partner, pull on the foot and ankle, stretching the leg on that side. This can be very pleasant for anyone who suffers from lower back pain. If you then go on to do the same with both feet at once the effect can be wonderful.

The lower leg can now receive some attention but I find that most people want only the most gentle of massaging here. In my opinion, long strokes are best and can be seen as a sort of foreplay to foot massage.

The feet Like the hands, the feet can be very responsive, if massaged properly. Indeed I have known many women to say that they feel nearly orgasmic when their feet are massaged. In Chapter Five, we look at reflexology and what this specific kind of foot massage has to offer but here let us look at ordinary, sensual foot massage.

Many people who are ticklish become somewhat apprehensive at the very thought of having their feet touched, let alone massaged for any length of time. But this is a quite unwarranted fear, if the giver knows what he or she is about. When massaging the feet, always use firm, big hand strokes. Start off by holding the foot between the flat of your hands and caressing it.

Now, gently but firmly pull the forefoot with one hand and, as this hand slides off the toes, grasp the foot again with the other hand and repeat the process. This "milking" movement provides fantastic sensations for most people. Repeat it several times, for each foot.

Now raise the foot with your hand and gently but firmly massage the sole just as you did the palm of the hand. Work around the area until you find the best places for the receiver, then concentrate on those. You will find that thumbs are best for this part of the foot massage. Do remember not to let your partner's foot simply fall back on to the floor. Set it down carefully before going on to the next foot.

Now pull the toes, one at a time, gently but firmly. Then run your fingertips through the spaces between the toes—as you did for the fingers. Lastly, hold and massage the whole foot.

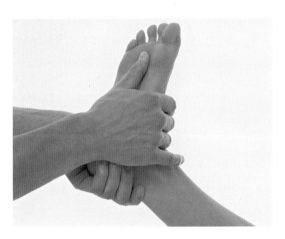

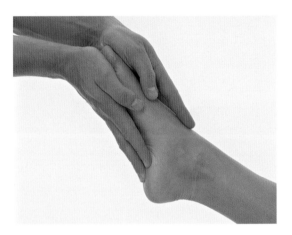

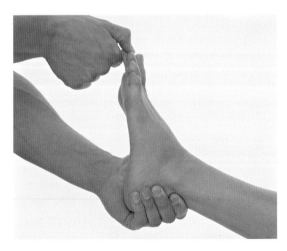

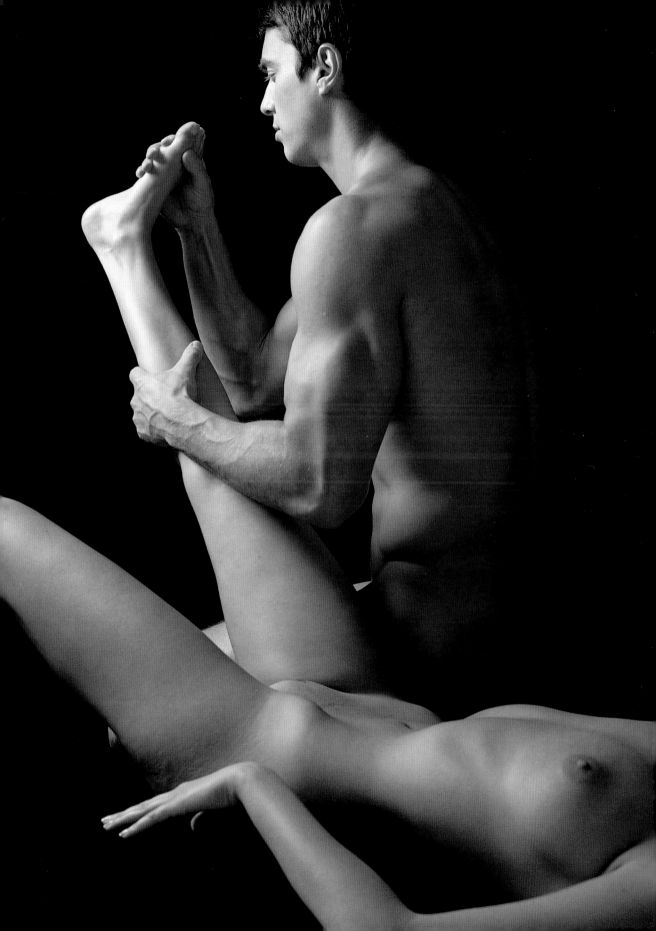

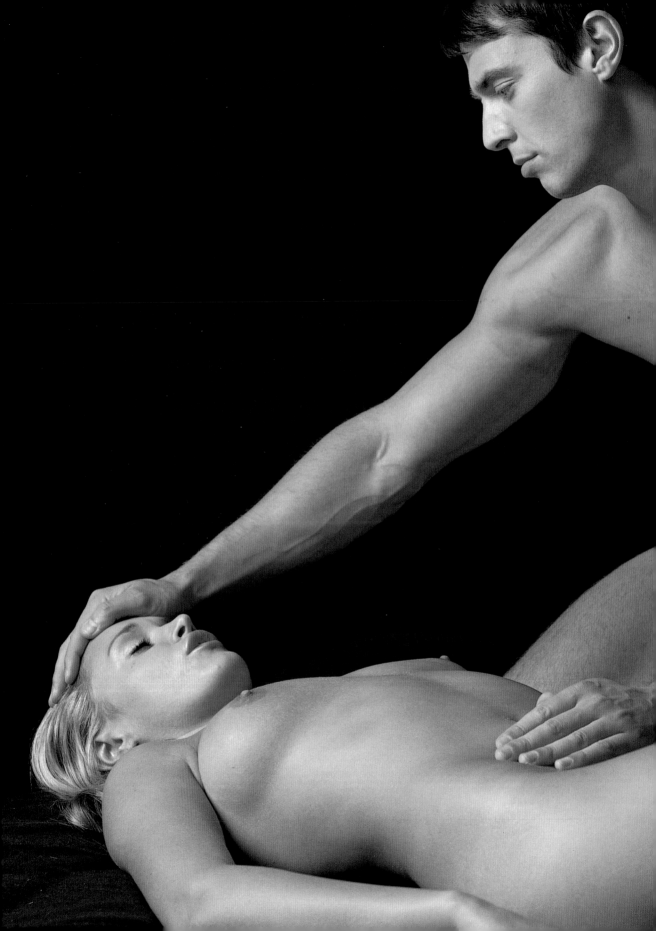

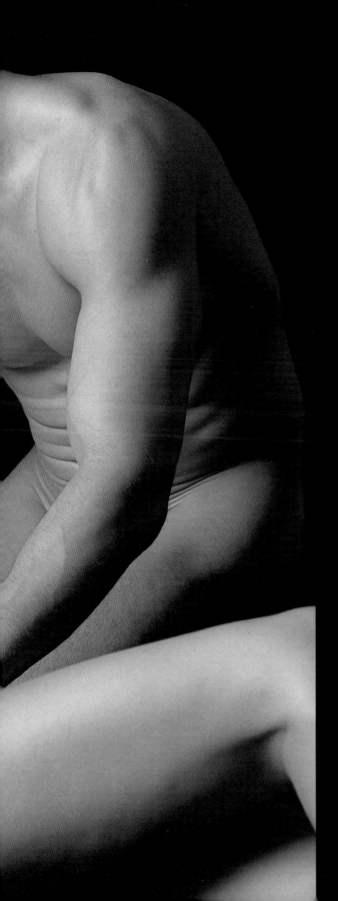

Finally—connection
Now you have completed all the separate areas of the body massage and your partner should be feeling very relaxed and may even have fallen asleep. End by connecting all the areas with some long, gentle strokes.

Sit or kneel at the side of the receiver and make long strokes with one hand up from one foot to the groin, across the lower stomach and down the other leg to the foot. Repeat this slowly and sensuously several times.

Now start just above the pubic area and run one hand up over the stomach and chest (around the breast) and down one arm, ending at the fingertips. Repeat this once more on this side and then do it twice more, but on the other side.

Finally, put one hand on your partner's forehead and the other on his or her stomach above the pubic area and just below the navel—and just sit peacefully for a minute or so while you finally connect up the energy patterns you have been making during the massage.

Now your partner can open his or her eyes and you can take things from here. Most people find that they are so relaxed that they simply want to cuddle and go to sleep. This is especially likely if they have chosen to do the massage at the end of the day.

You may, of course, feel exceptionally loving and close and want to show this by going on to erotic massage which may, or may not, end in orgasm for one or both of you.

The important thing about sensual massage is that it is not generally a form of foreplay. I have said this to many couples who have come back a week or two later to say that they got carried away and ended up having sex. This is all very fine but, in the long term, it defeats the purpose. If sensual massage is to be a pleasurable activity in itself then the receiver particularly has to be able to relax and feel totally at ease—trusting in the knowledge that there will be no price to pay at the end. I usually suggest that the partners agree not even to ask for sex on the first few occasions when they practice sensual massage. Once they see that the two can be separated and that a request for a massage does not have to end in sex, the two can be integrated as the weeks go by, perhaps using the further skills of erotic massage.

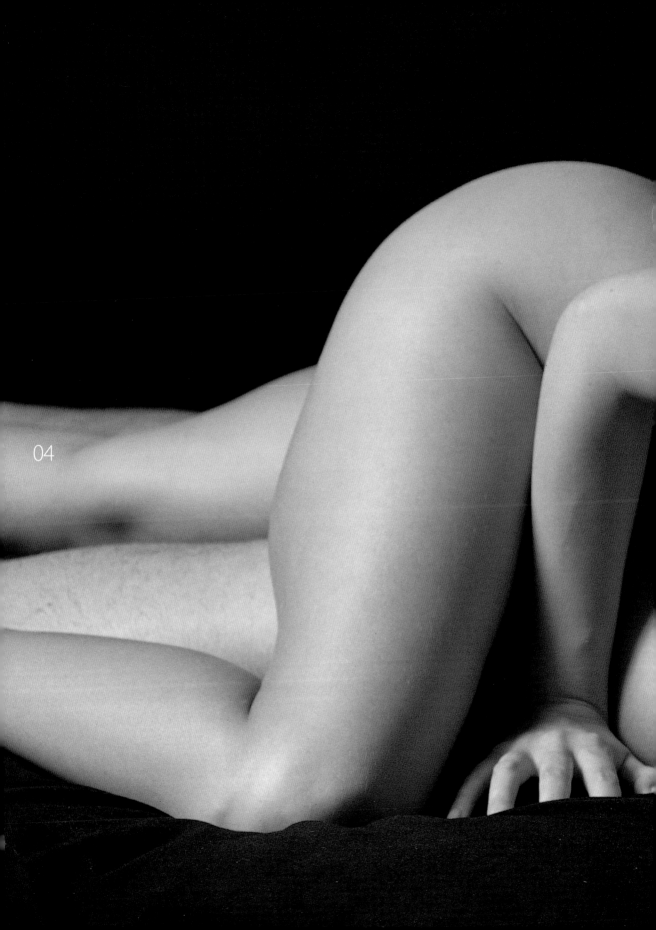

04

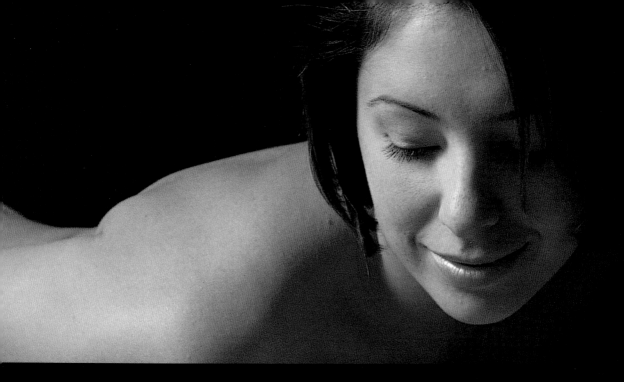

The joy of erotic massage

In the last chapter, we saw that sensual massage is designed to pleasure your partner without producing sexual arousal.

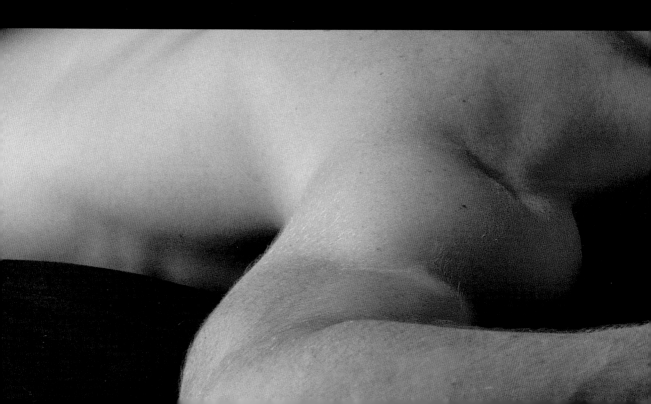

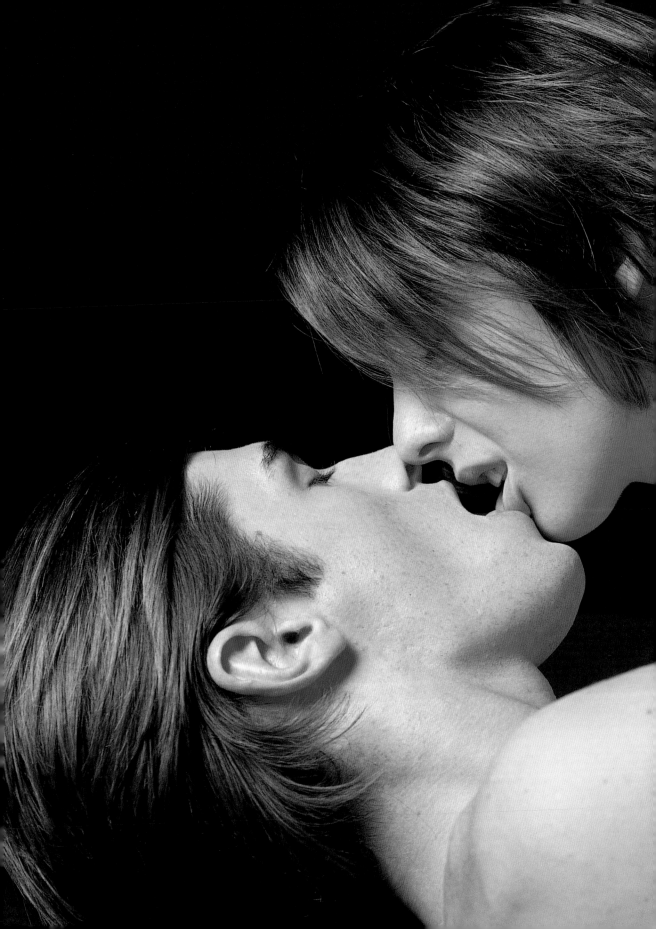

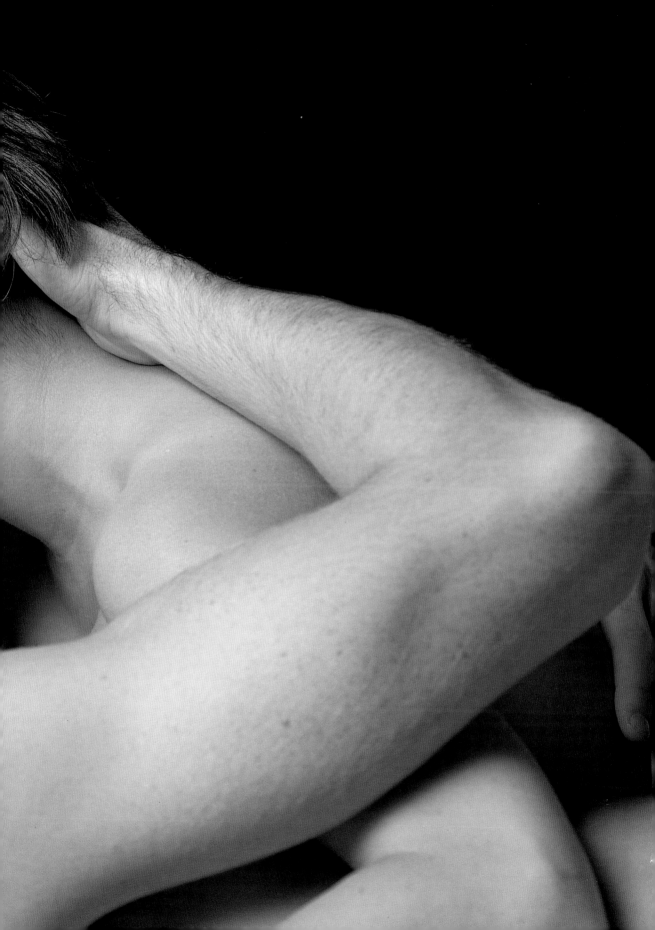

At first, many couples find this unlikely, but once they get used to the idea that they can give and receive physical pleasure without touching the genitals it alters their whole viewpoint—usually for the better.

What is erotic massage? Erotic massage is quite a different matter than sensual massage. Its aim is to arouse your partner as a prelude to sexual activity. The activity need not, of course, be full sexual intercourse. Some couples today, especially if they are not sure of one another's sexual past and are fearful of catching a sexually transmitted disease or getting pregnant, use erotic massage as a prelude to foreplay that ends in mutual masturbation. This is nothing new, of course; couples have always done this, especially where they have been unsure of their contraceptive safety.

The massage routine is totally different then, when it comes to erotic massage. Now the whole idea is to use your body and hands to arouse your partner, rather than produce relaxation and sensuous feelings. We will consider here only those techniques that stop short of masturbation because this subject is well covered by other books.

If we are to have any hope of arousing a partner by using erotic massage we must understand what kinds of massage turn them on. In order to do this, it helps to be aware which areas of the body are particularly sensitive to erotic massage and which are not. As we have already seen, almost the whole body benefits from sensual massage.

The erogenous zones The whole surface of our body is covered with nerve endings that transmit messages to the brain. But the whole body is not uniformly represented in the touch-sensitive areas of the brain; some areas have much more sensitivity than others.

While some areas are highly sensitive in relation to touch generally, others seem to have a specifically high erotic value, so that when they are stimulated they create a feeling of sexual arousal. As with everything to do with human sexuality the variations are great. Women, particularly, differ greatly in what they find erotic so a man will not necessarily be able to transfer experience learned from one woman to another.

Having said this, however, most people have in common some areas of their body that, when stimulated by the right person in the right way, cause them to become sexually aroused.

By and large, these areas are the "forbidden zones" that we avoid when socially touching others. We avoid such contact because these areas are so sensitive that we could evoke an inappropriate response.

As a couple gets to know each other the first erogenous zones to be discovered are the lips and the mouth. This takes us right back to babyhood when we experience so many pleasurable feelings through our mouth. A baby enjoys not only its mother's breast, its food, and its fingers, but also most of its toys, blankets, and a host of other things which it takes into its mouth as a highly efficient, early way of exploring them. The pleasures associated with oral lovemaking are highly enjoyable, relaxing and uninhibited and are thus of vital importance in erotic massage.

The next areas we discover are usually the face, ears and neck. These are anatomically close to the lips and mouth and are uncovered and therefore easily accessible when a couple are courting. The head and neck area is an excellent, nonthreatening place at which to start an erotic massage.

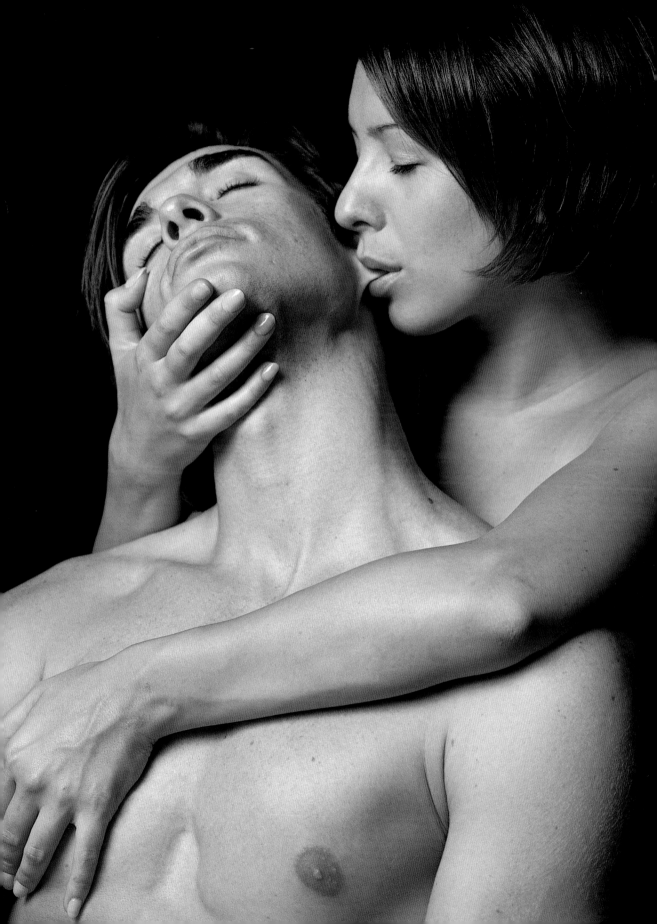

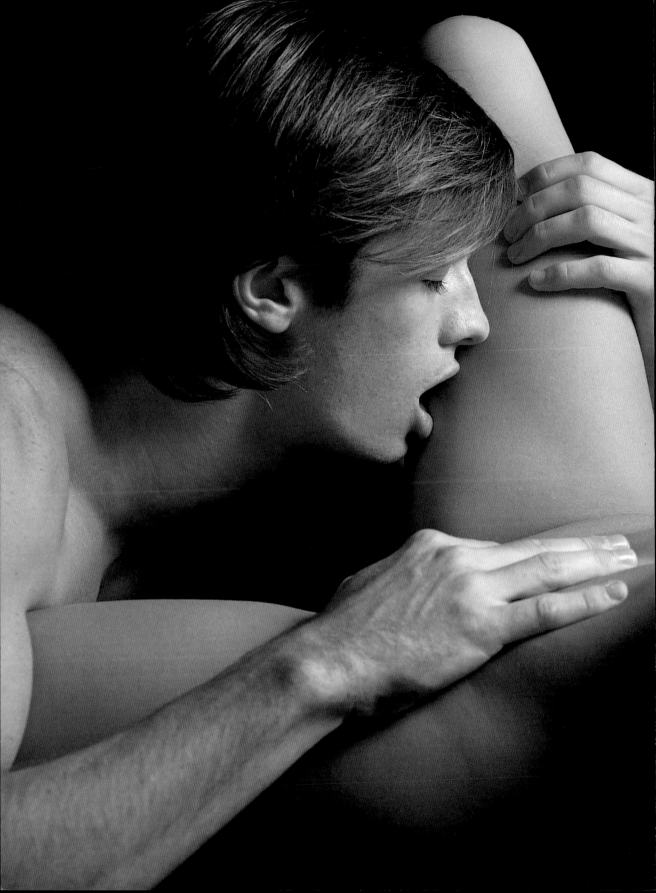

The inner surfaces of the thighs are sensitive, too, particularly in women. Indeed, some women become near-orgasmic when this area—perhaps in combination with the backs of their knees—is stroked or kissed.

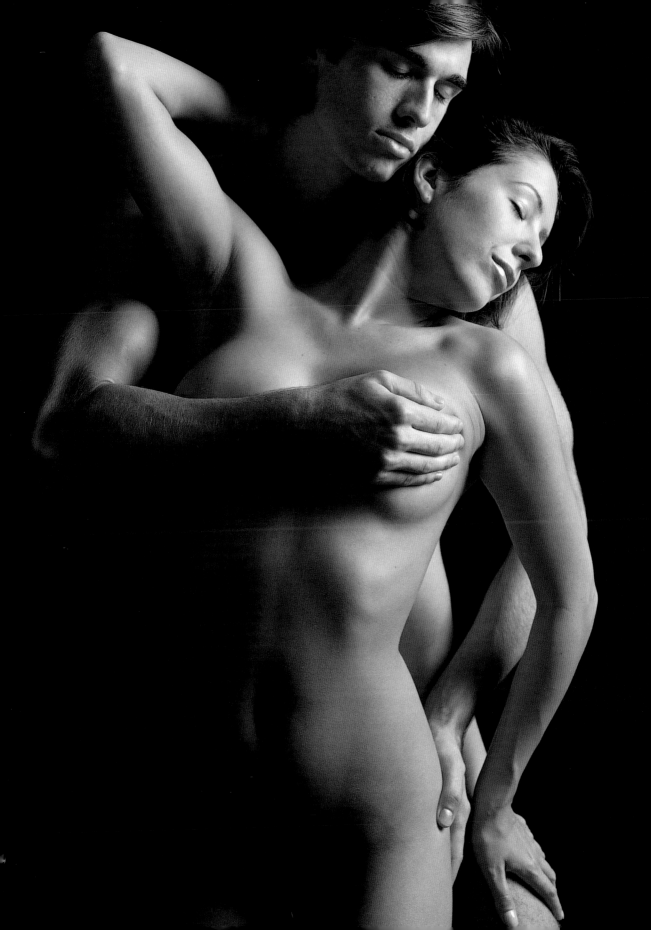

A woman's breasts can also be highly responsive of course, although about half of all women say that they are not as erotic as men imagine them to be. Far too many men turn their first attention to their partner's breasts and then wonder why she turns away. At least early on, while they are still becoming aroused, most women simply prefer to have their breasts gently held and caressed. Later they might enjoy other things (see page 91). This raises an important issue in relation to erotic massage: What feels good at one stage might well not at another, and vice versa. This makes erotic massage rather different from sensual massage in that the latter is much more predictable, partly because it does not rely on any emotional or sexual chemistry between the couple. Erotic massage, by definition, involves the intimate personalities of the couple as lovers and this means that the whole pursuit is more subject to the uniqueness of the individuals and to the state of their relationship at that time.

All of the anatomical areas so far discussed are known as the "secondary erogenous zones." The "primary erogenous zones" are the penis, scrotum and perineal area in men and the equivalent area in women, which is called the vulva. We shall not be considering these in this book because there are many other publications that deal with stimulation of these areas.

Generally, women are more responsive to touch than are men. This is because they have more pleasure zones than men have. Women are also more at ease with their bodies and feel free to experience pleasure from them more readily than do most men. Boys are brought up to be tough and to deny their feelings and consequently many men find it hard to relax and even to acknowledge their pleasurable sensations, unless, of course, they are genital. Men come to believe that the only "real" sexual activity they should indulge in and enjoy is genital activity and that anything else is a waste of time, or "feminine."

For these reasons, while most women greatly enjoy erotic massage that excludes the genitals, men are eager, or even frankly impatient, to get on with "the real thing." This would be no tragedy in itself if men married men but they do not. Many women complain that their partners lack sensitivity and patience—going straight for the genitals as if nothing else mattered.

This is perhaps not too surprising given the way boys are reared to be "men" in our culture, but it is also encouraged by the fact that for most men their best erotic sensations occur in the area covered by their underwear. This is not so for women; women have a much greater area over which they enjoy being stimulated. In fact, some women can be brought to orgasm by the stimulation of almost any part of their anatomy. This certainly could not be said of men.

While almost any part of the body can be touched, stroked, massaged, or kissed during an erotic massage, for best effect it makes sense to concentrate on those areas of your partner's body that you have found from experience to be erogenous. Having said this, men often need encouragement and "tutoring" if they are really to enjoy being massaged erotically. They assume that their erogenous zones are few in number—and well-known to them—and so miss out on many others that could be developed with practice. But a woman who is enthusiastic, willing and inventive will find ways to delight her partner, however un-erotic he thinks himself to be at the start.

Some basic skills Let us now look at
some basic techniques for lovers to use
when doing an erotic massage, just as we
did when looking at sensual massage. Here,
as then, it is important to remember that
these are only suggestions and that you will
find your own special methods as you
become more adventurous and skilled.

At first, most people think of erotic massage as
involving only manual skills but it can include far
more as we shall see. Whatever technique you use,
the thing to remember is that the slower you go and
the more you tease the better the effects you will
achieve. Erotic massage has nothing in common with
quickie sex—delicious though that might be at the
right time. Erotic massage techniques prolong lovemaking by means of erotic touch until both of you
are so crazy with passion for one another that you
cannot bear to delay intercourse for a second longer.
　　Here then, are some basic techniques and skills
that are worth trying and practicing.

Use your hands
Erotic massage is very different from the sensual
variety because here the sole purpose is to arouse
your partner and there are no holds barred. No longer
do you have to stifle your natural desire to become
intensely involved because your intimate involvement
is the key to success.
　　In the next section, we will look at each area of
the body and how to massage it specifically for the
greatest erotic effect but here let us look at some of
the basic strokes.

Gliding is particularly erotic. Run your hands over
large areas of your partner's body, especially the back,
chest and breasts, buttocks and spine. It is not
necessary to oil your partner for this but if you have
just completed a sensual massage he or she will
already he slightly lubricated. Make the strokes long
and integrating rather than short and jerky. Start by
letting your hands "float" over the surface of the
receiver's body and when breaking the stroke do
so gently and sensitively.

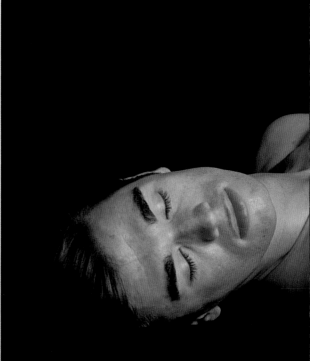

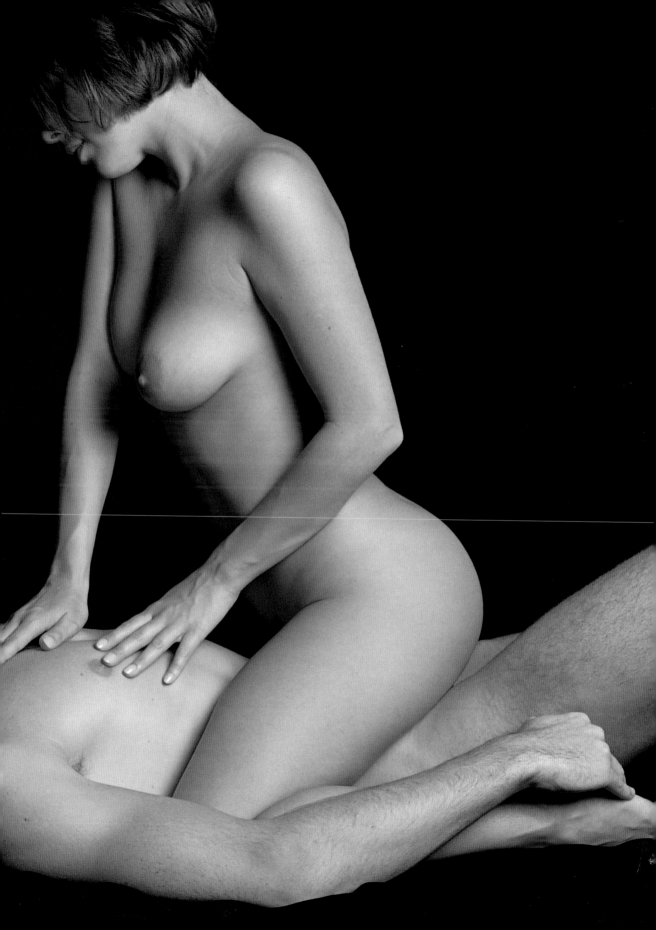

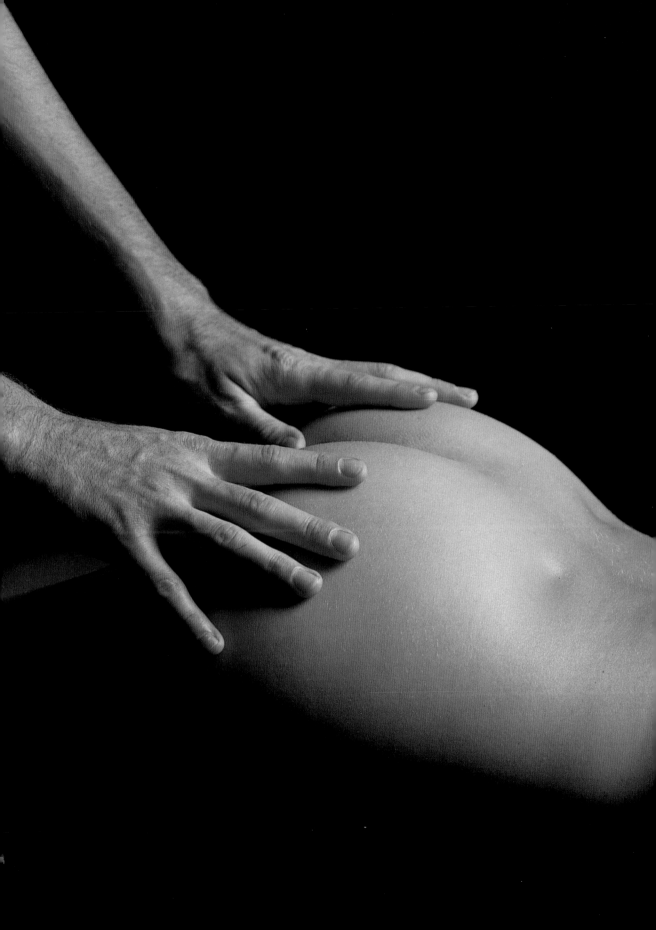

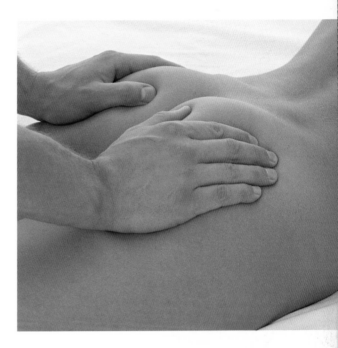

Kneading and other semi-deep strokes can be very erotic in the right places. Some people find that, once they begin to become aroused, areas of tension such as the top of the back around the shoulders and the base of the neck can be exquisitely erotic if the amount of pressure applied is just right. By and large, though, deep and semi-deep strokes are best reserved for your sensual massage.

Light touching, using your fingers as lightly as if they were spider's legs, is highly arousing. Let your hands wander all over your partner's body just touching the skin's surface with your fingertips in a teasing, not tickling, way. Explore further wherever it makes them shudder with delight. Almost anywhere is good to try. Trace long paths linking areas that you learn are responsive. We are avoiding the genital area for the purposes of this book but just a warning here that these spider's legs strokes are too ticklish for most people's genitals.

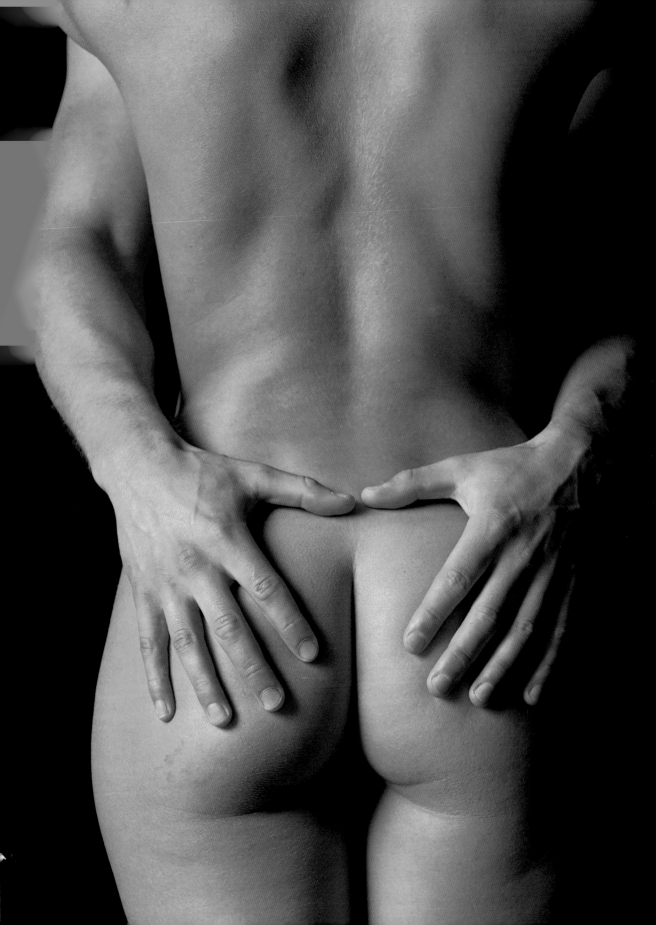

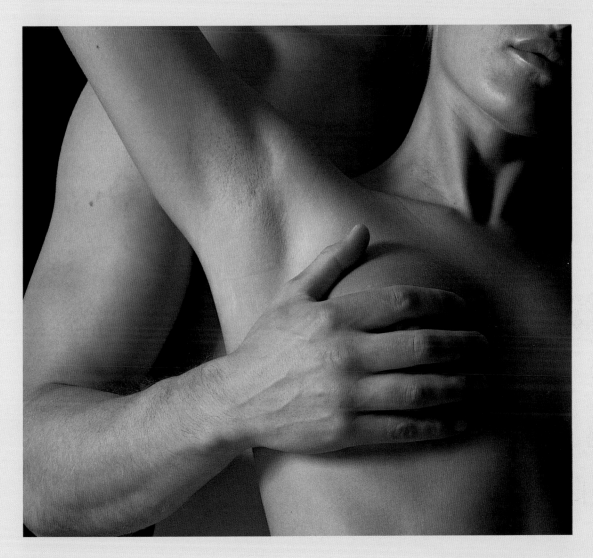

Walking your fingertips around various sensitive parts can be a delight and gentle **pinching** and **squeezing** can be good, if done in the right places—that is, the fleshy parts of the body.

As your partner becomes highly aroused he or she might enjoy actually being squeezed hard. This is true of some women's breasts and indeed some men's nipples. Many people like to have their buttocks squeezed and, of course, a whole body hug can make you feel very close indeed. Some couples who become very close emotionally during their erotic massage say that they occasionally feel that they want their bodies to merge into one another, so deep is the intimacy that they feel.

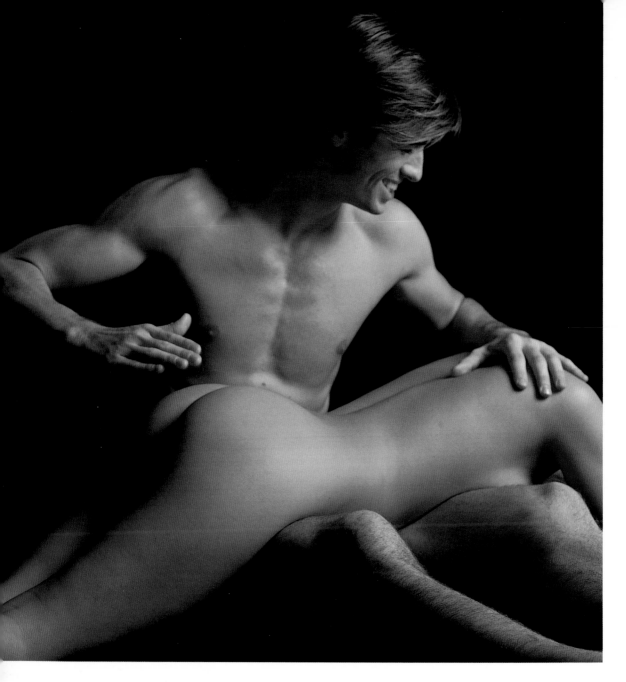

Smacking is a rather specialized form of stroke but one which is enjoyed by some. Indeed, there are women who need to be smacked, playfully, before they can truly enjoy the sex that is to follow. This is probably because they are unconsciously guilty about enjoying, or even wanting, sex and feel that they should be punished in advance for being so "naughty." It is a foolish lover who does not include such play if it turns his partner on.

Of course you don't have to limit yourself to using your hands to massage your partner's body where he

or she best enjoys intimate contact. At first this might feel a little strange but as you become used to it you will become very skilled and give your partner sensations that he or she never knew were possible.

In fact, a fun game to play is to forbid the use of hands altogether and see how inventive, erotic, and sensual you can be without their help.

Remember that whatever you do, and however you achieve it, the only goal is to give your partner the best erotic sensations and to drive him or her to higher levels of passion.

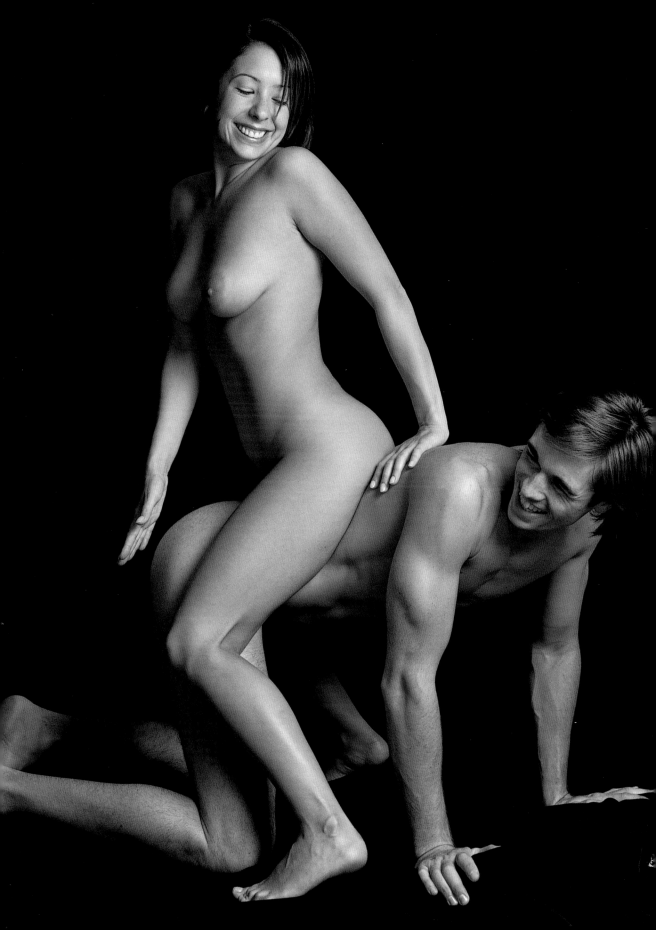

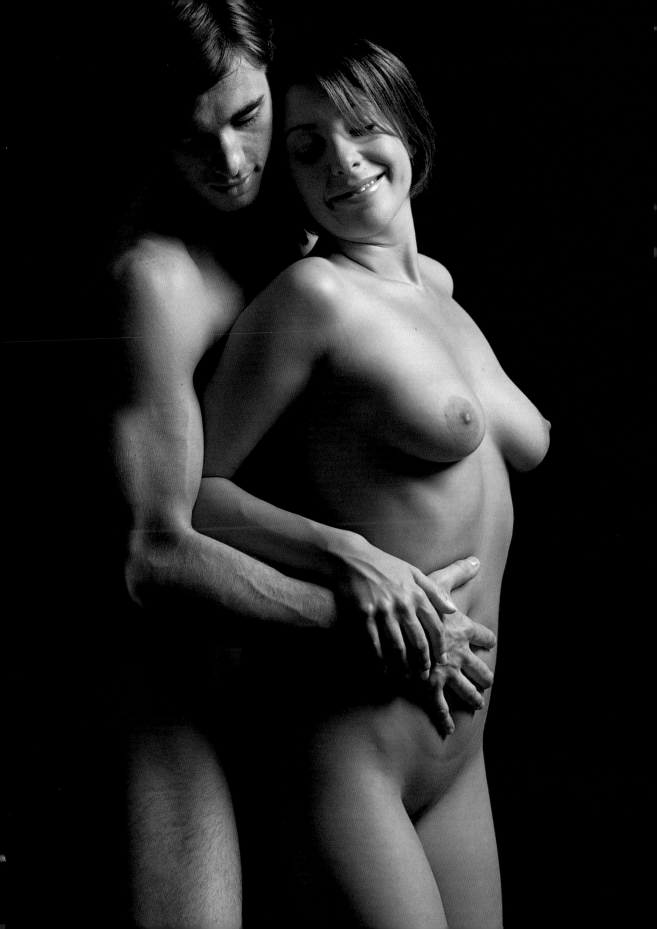

Use your hair

A very erotic thing for a woman to do is to let her hair trail over various sensitive areas of the man's body. The gentle, teasing nature of this form of "massage" is hard to beat.

Use your mouth

Obviously you will want to kiss your partner's erogenous zones but there are many other mouth games you can play, too. Run your tongue around sensitive areas in a teasing but non-tickling way; give your partner little nibbles and nips with your teeth— but taking care not to hurt him or her. Blow puffs of air over highly sensitive areas. Suck an area of skin into your mouth and work your tongue on it. The combinations are endless.

Some couples enjoy using their tongues to "bathe" one another. Make sure that your tongue is wet with saliva, then run it all over areas of your partner's body as if you were washing it with your tongue. Blowing dry air over these wetted areas can be exquisite for the receiver.

As a part of this tongue bath, or maybe separately, don't forget to kiss your partner's body really erotically. Kissing the palm of the hand, for example, can be very sensual; kiss the fingers too and perhaps take them into your mouth one at a time. In other words, extend your ideas of kissing from simply planting your lips on your partner's skin to becoming a way of oral lovemaking in every sense of the word. Oral sex has come to be seen as a very narrow business involving one partner kissing or sucking the genitals of the other but this misses out a whole range of wonderful sensations, many of which are highly erotic.

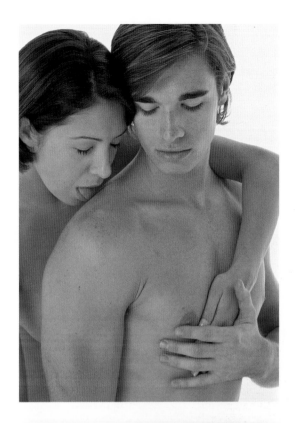

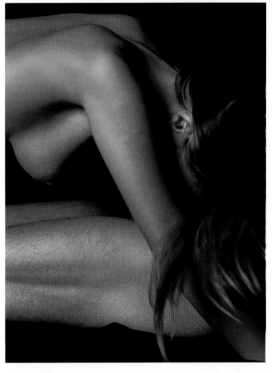

If you are a woman, use your breasts

Either ask your partner to oil your breasts or, alternatively, smooth a little oil over the area of his body you intend to massage and then use your breasts to massage him there. This drives most men wild and often has a similar effect on the woman. Using your breasts to massage his nipples can be especially erotic.

In addition to this extensive repertoire you could also go back to any of the strokes or techniques that you found produced erotic effects when doing your sensual massage. Instead of reducing the erotic effect as you did then the idea now is to enhance it.

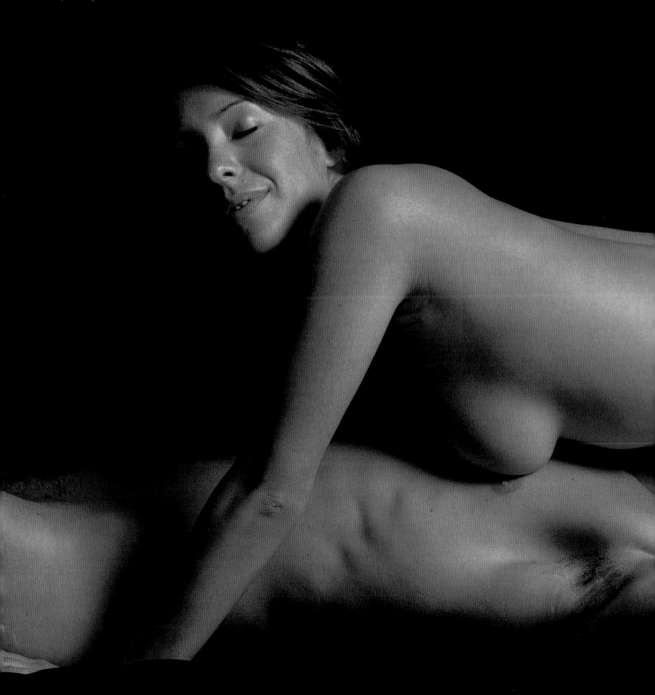

Use your mind

The mind is our most powerful sex organ and the skin is the largest, so between the two, it is easy to see that erotic massage is a very powerful and arousing pastime, involving them both.

Really concentrate on your partner. Your practice with the sensual massage will come in handy here. Don't work out the shopping list or let worries about the mortgage clutter your mind—lose yourself in the present activity and give your partner the best sensations you can. He or she will be doing the same for you so, if you have built up some tension and expectation as a result of your sensual massage, now is the time to defuse it.

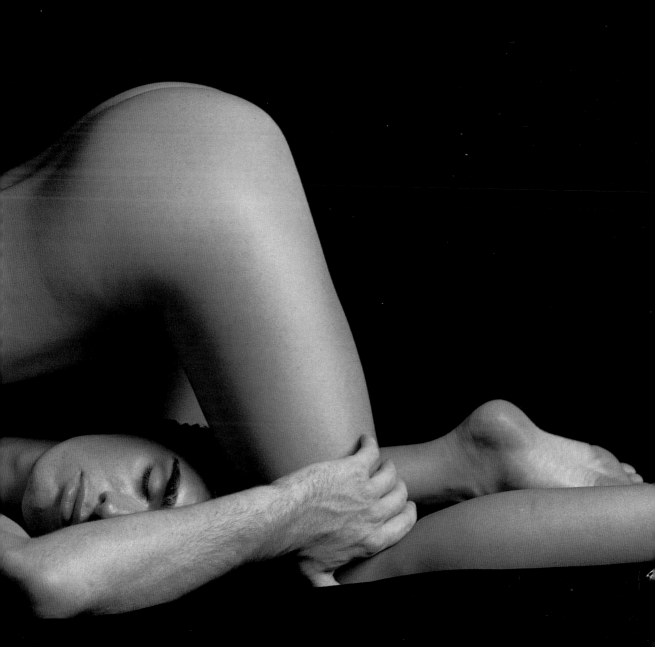

Use toys and aids

Electrical massagers, feathers, furs, ice, silk, leather, rubber, and a host of other material aids can be used to enhance the erotic quality of the massage. It's fun experimenting with these in order to increase your repertoire and enjoyment.

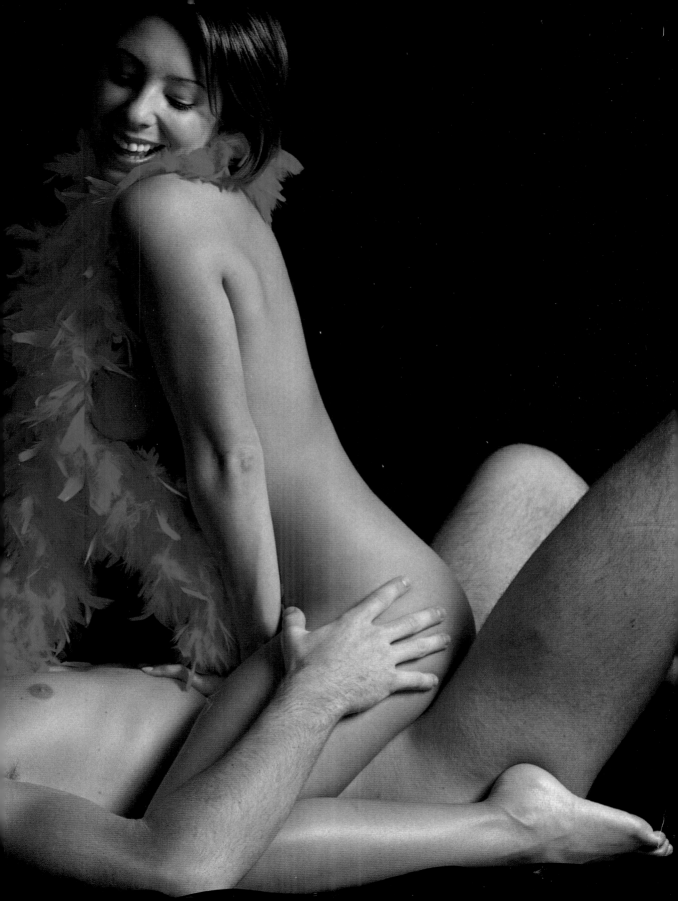

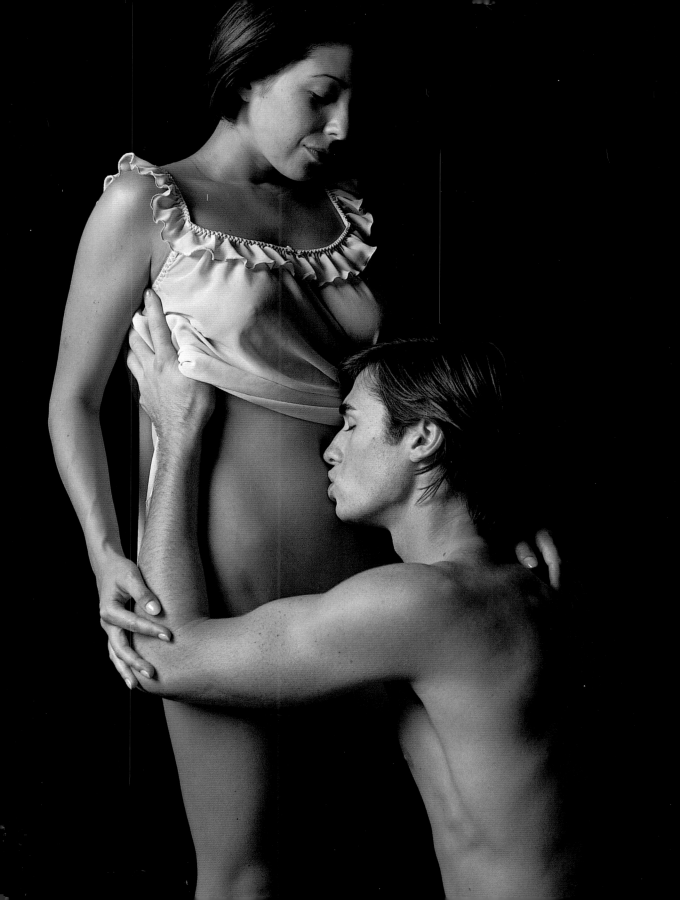

Setting the scene
How you set the scene for erotic massage depends somewhat on whether or not it is to be a follow-up from sensual massage.

If you are following up from sensual massage then you will already have made your environment conducive to relaxation and not being disturbed. The only difference now perhaps is that you might want to go to the bed rather than stay on the massage mat or floor. You will by now be intent on more uninhibited sharing and the firmness of the floor will probably be uncomfortable for cuddling and anything that follows.

However, if you are starting out to give each other an erotic massage without these preliminaries then look back to page 16 to see which of the preparations listed there and on the following pages apply to your plans for an erotic encounter. Some things will be more important to get right and others less so. For example, privacy, while important when massaging each other sensually is vital when doing erotic massage. Few people can become sufficiently uninhibited to really enjoy themselves erotically if they fear interruption.

Some couples like to enhance the mood of the room for erotic occasions, perhaps by putting on some music that has a special romantic or erotic significance for them.

Clothes, while definitely not a part of sensual massage, can play an important role in erotic massage. Many men enjoy their partner being dressed up in a special dress or underwear and some women obtain pleasure from their man dressing in particular ways. Undressing then becomes an integral part of the massage and one part of the body can be revealed at a time and worked on as a prolonged tease.

It is fine to wear jewelry provided that it does not get in the way. Perfume also adds to the erotic atmosphere.

How you prepare your body and that of your partner is also more important than for sensual massage. Bathing or showering together is a good start, in fact it is nice to begin the massage in a shared shower or bath.

Mental preparation is just as important as it is for sensual massage except that now, instead of stilling your mind and focusing on your partner's pleasure, you excite your mind, perhaps by fantasizing a favorite scene. Some couples further enhance this by sexy talk.

All of this preparation raises the level of sexual expectation and tension and extends the amount of time and pleasure you will derive from the massage itself. In a hectic world in which many couples hurry through their lovemaking as if it were a meal in a fast-food restaurant, this leisurely approach pays dividends and can even completely revive an ailing sex life.

Couples often ask me whether or not they should do a sensual massage before starting on their erotic massage. Frankly there's no simple answer to this because some people find that they usually end up making love after they have massaged one another sensually and others never do. Obviously, erotic massage is sufficient in itself and does not have to follow or be a part of a sensual massage. I still think it is valuable to separate the two pursuits on most occasions so that the person asking for a massage doesn't have to expect to pay for it by having to go on to sex if they do not want to do so. Obviously, this is not a problem when it comes to erotic massage because sex is intended from the start.

The main thing that most couples who practice both these techniques find is that they become much more honest with one another about what they really want. Too often a man who feels in need of a cuddle or a back rub after a long drive home from work thinks he has to clothe his request in some sort of sexual language or his partner will think him a wimp. He therefore asks for sex when really he wants something else. Because his heart (and his penis) are not in it he is more prone to failure and this, added to the fact that it wasn't really sex that he wanted in the first place, leads to disappointments, failures, rows, bitterness, and even perhaps to an extramarital search by one or both partners to vent their frustration.

If as a result of asking for what they want, and being sure that they will receive it, a couple becomes more open about what it is that they do want, then massaging one another greatly enhances the relationship. Women too, often find it difficult to be honest. Sometimes a woman goes along with sex when she really would rather not, but had she offered

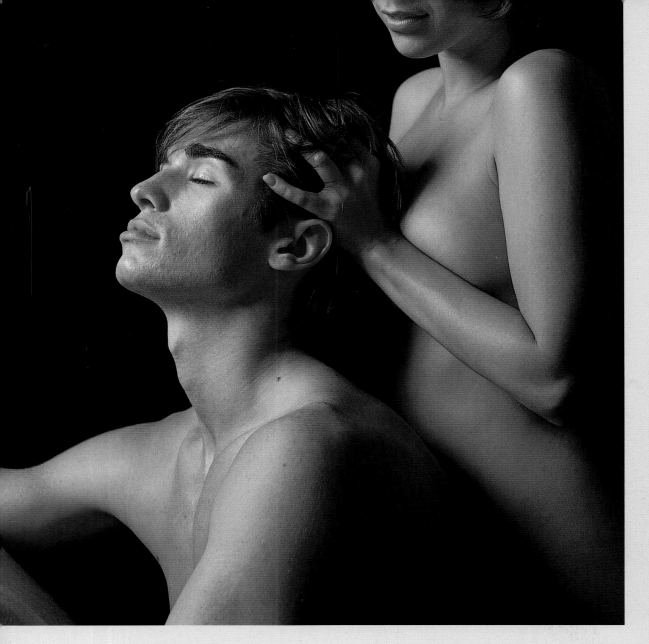

her man a sensual massage or even a stimulating erotic one followed by masturbation both would be happy and she would not end up feeling put upon.

Some couples make deals with one another in this sphere of their lives and who is to say that they are wrong? For example, the woman may be feeling sexy but the man may be too tired for intercourse. Or he may have had a recent failure and be wary of things going wrong again. Such a man might, however, be happy to settle for an erotic massage, with or without masturbation. It is nonthreatening and because his partner is being so uninhibitedly arousing to him he

doesn't feel so bad about "letting her down" by not having sex.

The permutations and combinations of sensual massage, erotic massage, masturbation, and intercourse are numerous and any thoughtful couple who want to please one another will work out a plan that suits them on any particular occasion. With flexibility and good will on both sides there are few sexual and intimate situations that cannot be dealt with lovingly, using a combination of sensual and erotic massage.

Erotic things to do
Any couple prepared to be adventurous will discover for themselves what they best enjoy but here I list a few of the things that many couples have found to work. This list is just a start; an uninhibited couple will easily be able to double it over some months of pleasuring one another.

Hair and scalp
Massage your partner's scalp and head, especially over tense muscles at the temples or at the back of the head. This can he a good soothing start because it is so relaxing. As we saw on page 60, the head and neck are also easily accessible (because they are not covered by clothes) and are areas of the body we are used to having petted from very early in life. This makes them a soothing, nonthreatening place at which to begin.

- Nuzzle your face into the hair and run your fingers through it repeatedly as you stroke your partner's scalp.
- Some women enjoy having a little perfume massaged into their scalp.
- Kiss each other's hair.
- Some people like to have their hair brushed by their partner in a rhythmical and sensual way. This can be very erotic in the right setting.

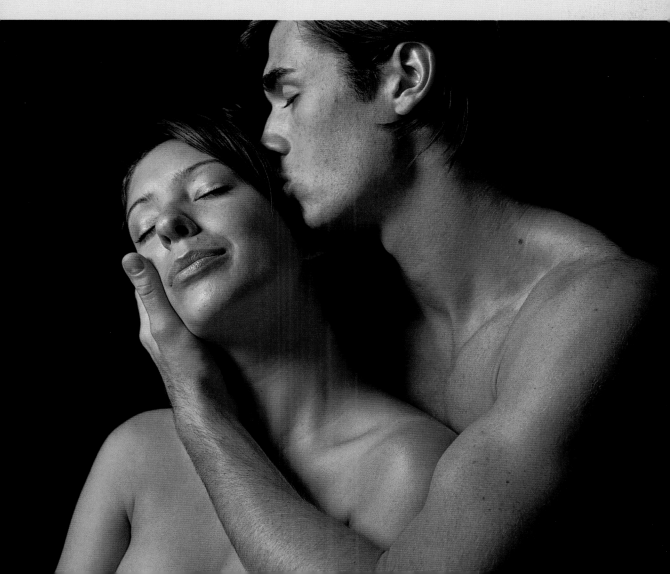

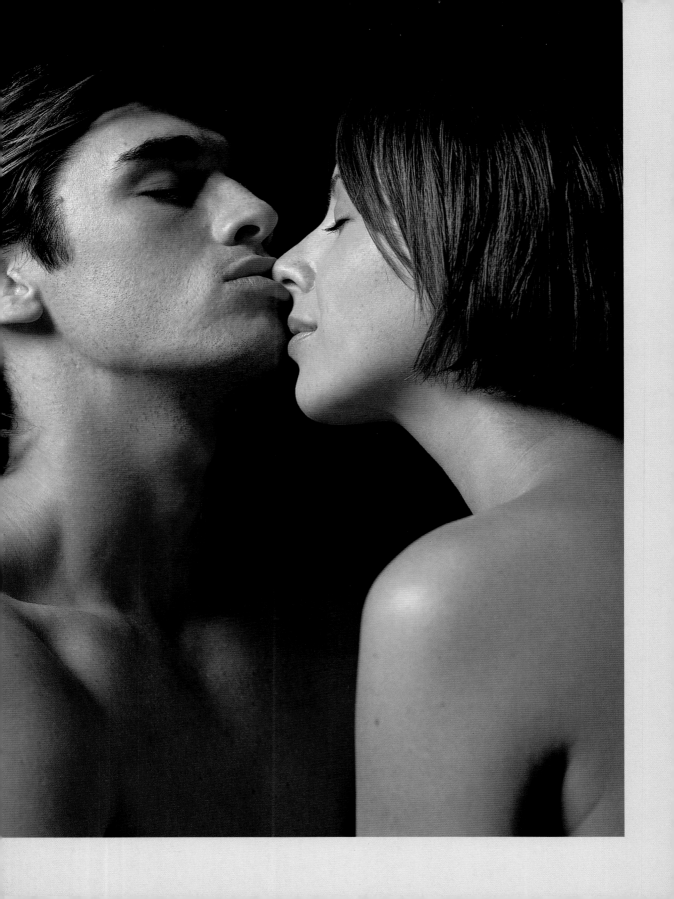

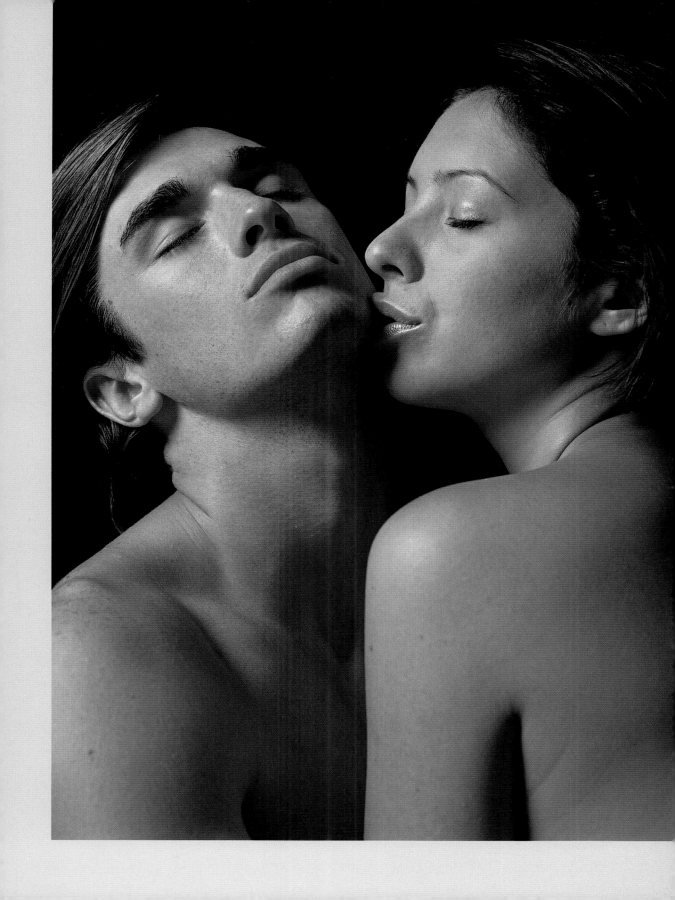

Face and ears

Kiss your partner's face all over and hold it in your hands, gently and lovingly.

- Plant masses of tiny and light kisses on various parts of the face, especially on the eyelids, and the ears.
- Touch the inside of the ear lobe, very lightly and sensuously, and trace paths around the outside too.
- Brush the lobe of the ear with a fingertip and gently bite it. Massage the ear with your tongue.
- Now gently run a fingertip over the eyelids; touch the lips; make tiny circles over the cheeks; and so on.
- Kiss each other on the lips and mouth using all the erotic skills you have learned during your time together.

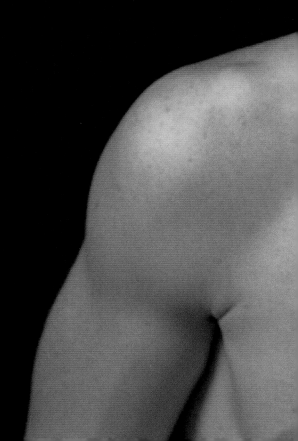

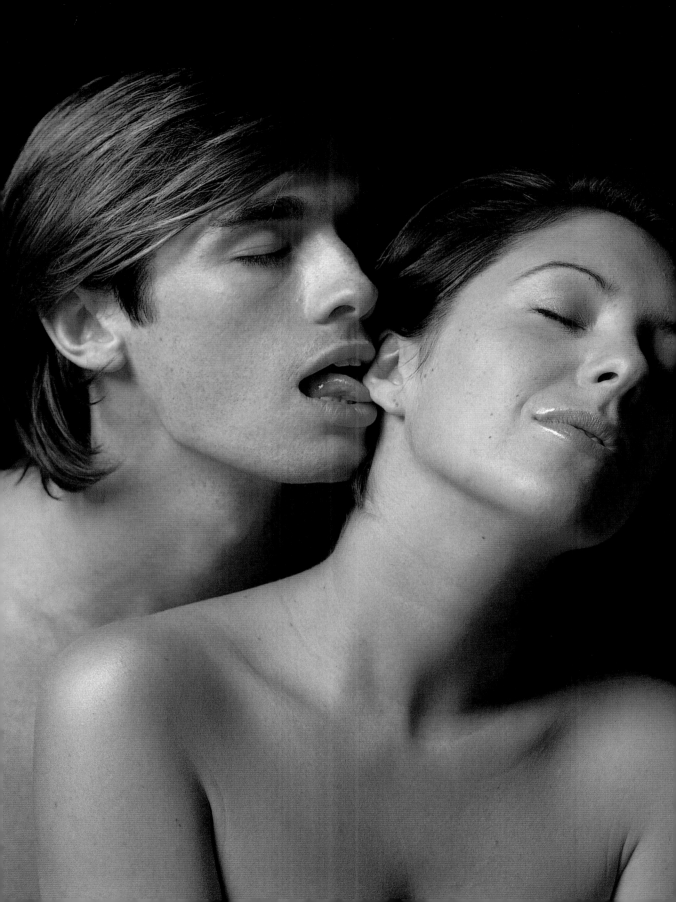

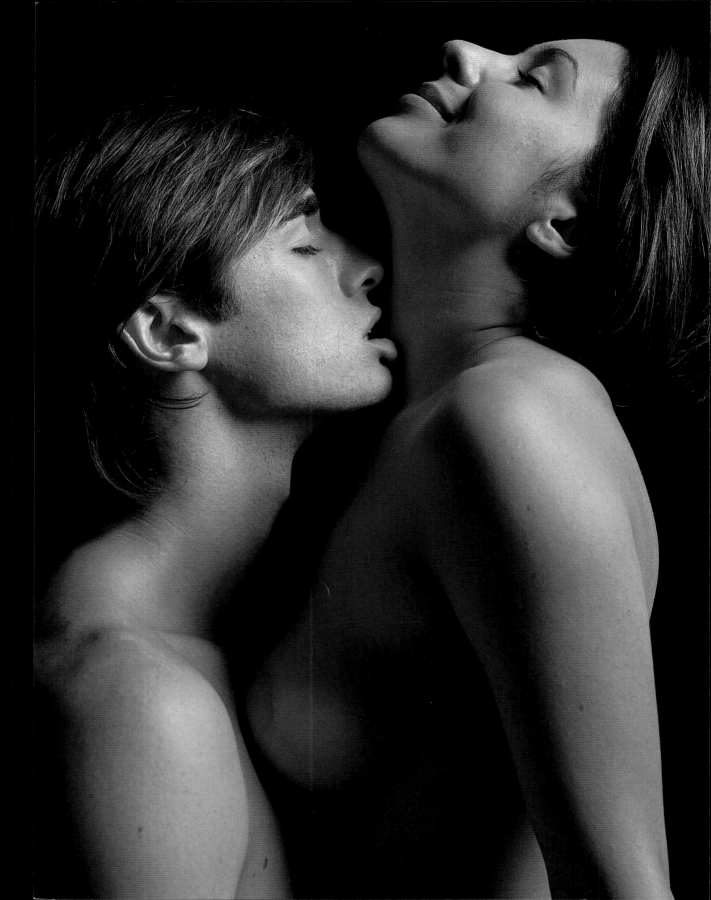

Neck

Stroke the sides of the neck with several fingertips bunched together.

- Breathe onto your partner's neck so that he or she feels the gentle warmth of your breath.
- Run your hands under the hairline and stroke the back of the neck with your fingertips.
- Bring your hands round to the front and gently trace a path along the collarbone.
- Plant kisses on your partner's throat, working from the top of the breastbone up to the tip of the chin. Repeat this up and down several times.

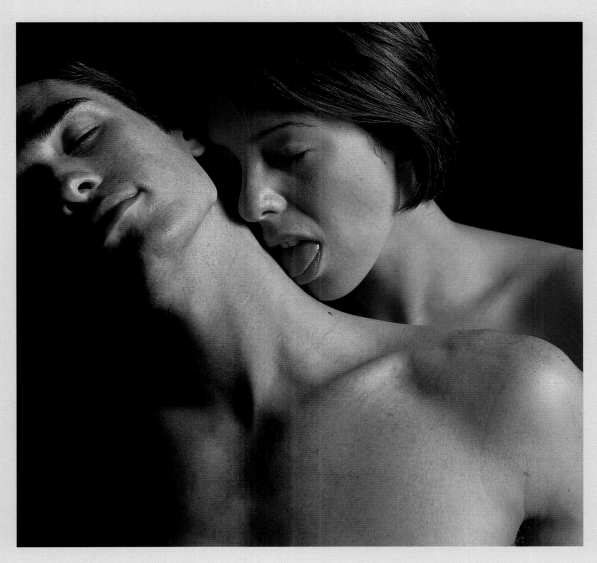

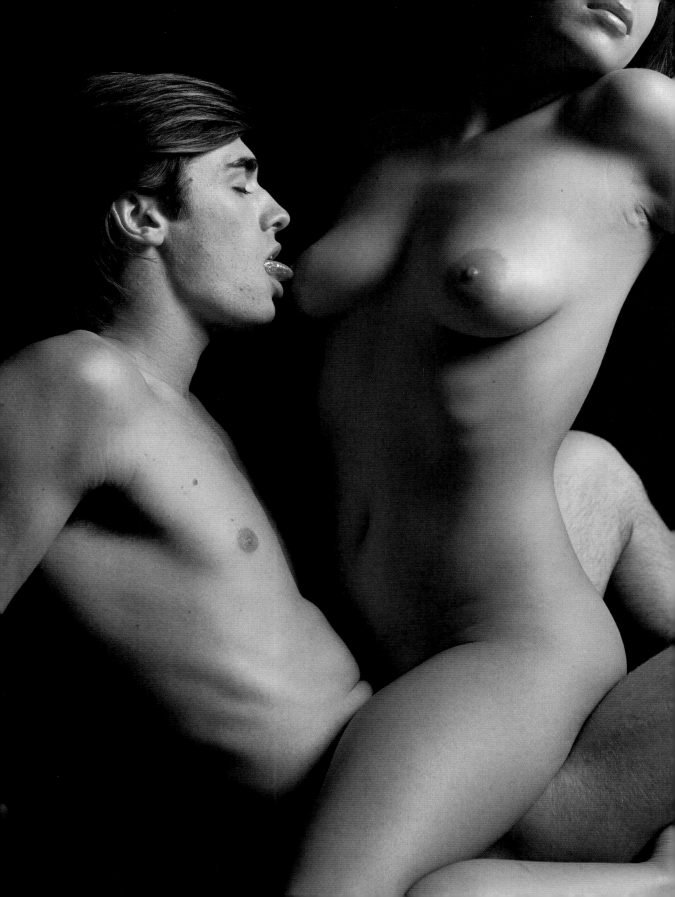

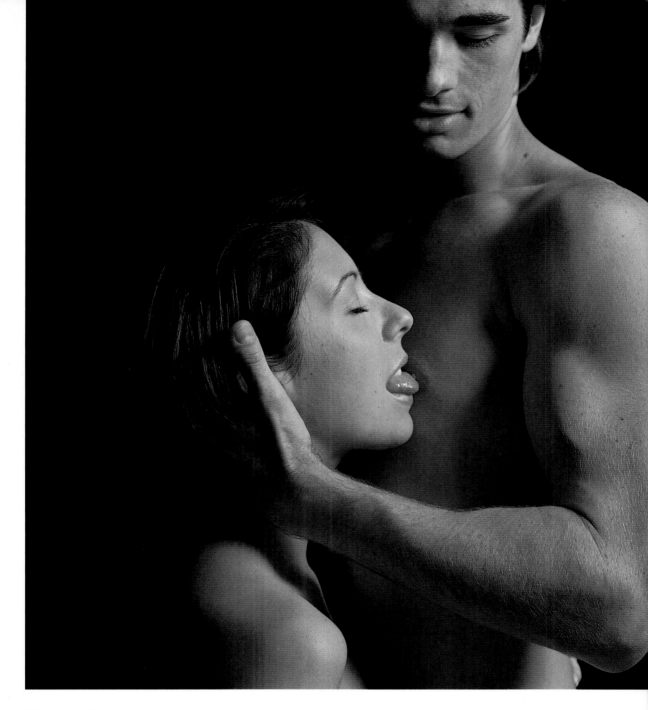

Chest and breasts

For him   Circle his nipples with your tongue and give them gentle, teasing bites. Stroke his chest all over, perhaps with some sensuous material such as silk. Rub your body over his chest, perhaps massaging his chest with your breasts through the silk.

Experiment until you discover what drives him wild. This may take some time because most men have little or no experience of what they best like done to this area of their bodies.

For her   This is not so for women, many of whom play with their breasts when masturbating and are thus quite expert on the subject of what turns them on. A sensible man watches his partner masturbate so that he knows exactly what she best likes and how she does it.

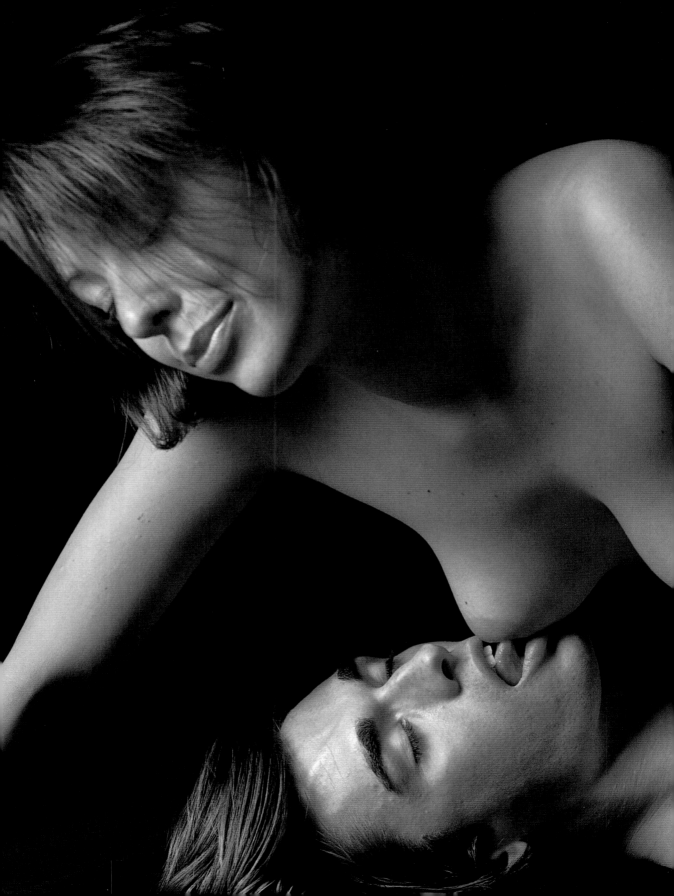

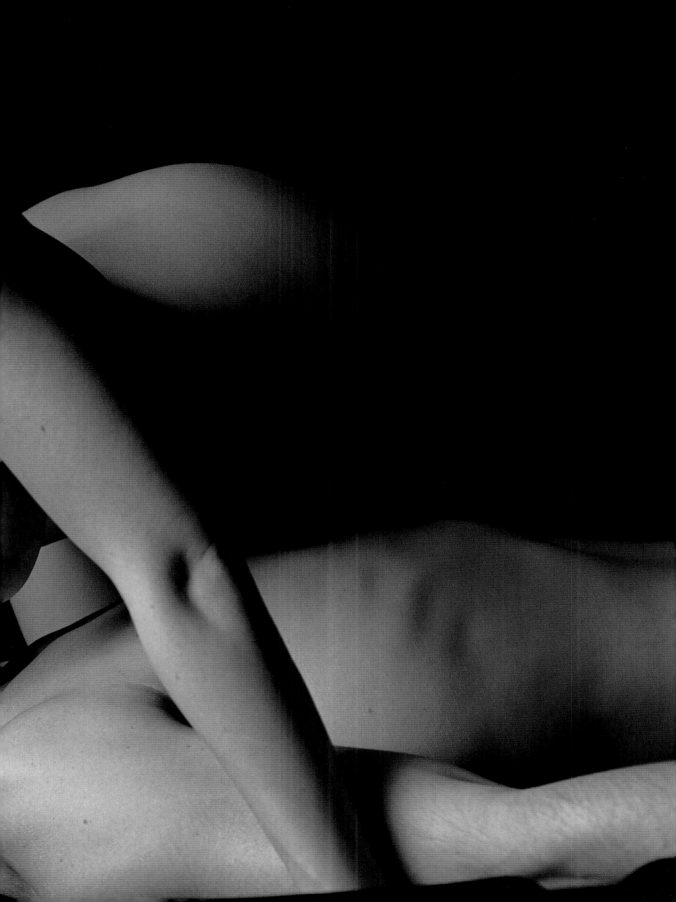

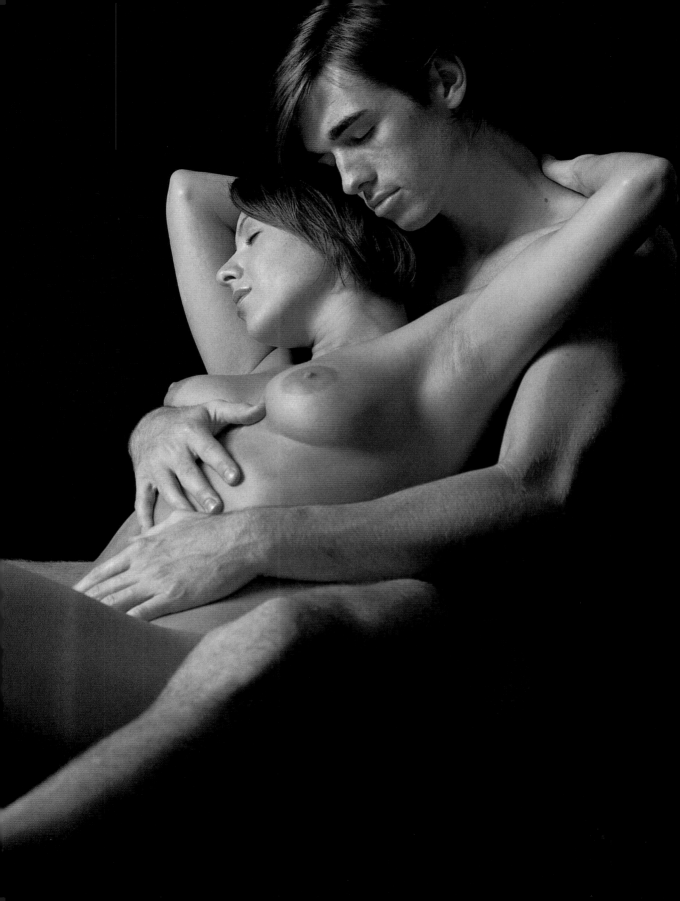

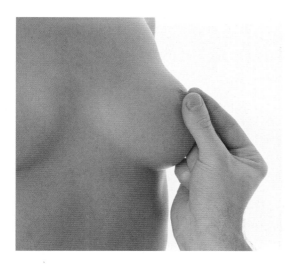

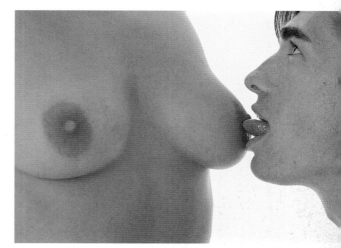

- Use the palm of your hand to brush lightly over her breasts (use some oil if you both want to massage her properly). Apply the oil all over the breasts and the top of her chest. Apply it slowly and teasingly leaving the nipples until last.
- Gently rub the nipples between your fingers. Squeeze them if this is what she likes. Push them into the breast itself and massage them in this position. Gently pull the nipples, perhaps slightly twisting them at the same time.
- Take as much of the breast into your mouth as you can and suck hard. Apply various kinds of suction to the nipples, at the same time tonguing them. When playing with one breast in this way, be sure to stroke the other one at the same time.

- Wet her nipples with saliva and blow softly on them.
- Grasp both breasts at once and gently rub them together.
- Cover her breasts with some pleasant food or drink and lick it off.
- Flutter your eyelashes over her nipples or use a feather.
- Rub your nipples against hers.
- Massage her breasts with your feet.

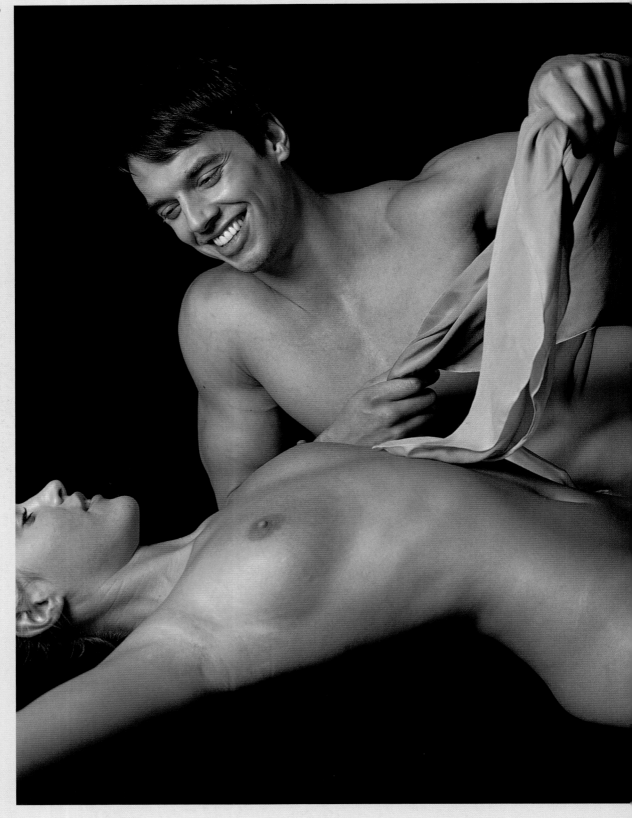

Stomach

Use a sensuous material to stroke your partner's
stomach. Silk underwear or stockings, especially if she
has just taken them off, can be a really erotic experience.
Kiss the whole of the stomach right down to the pubic
hair but teasingly refrain from actually touching it.
*   Put your tongue into the navel and rotate it. Now
    blow into the navel.

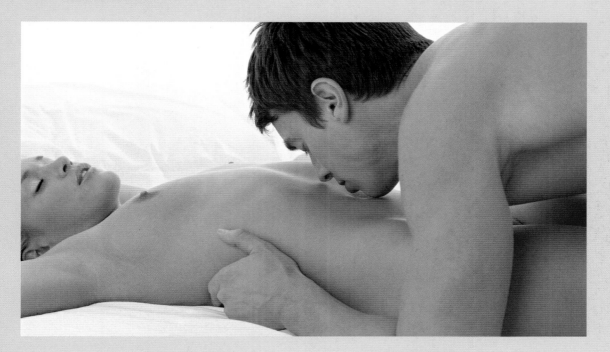

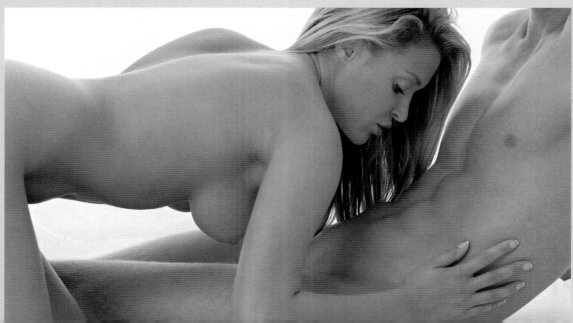

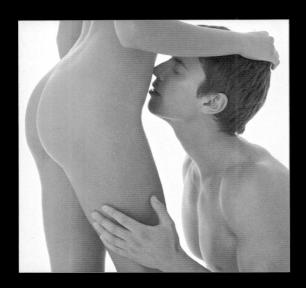

- Cover the stomach with hot breaths.
  While doing any of these things, keep your hands
  busy caressing another part of the body.

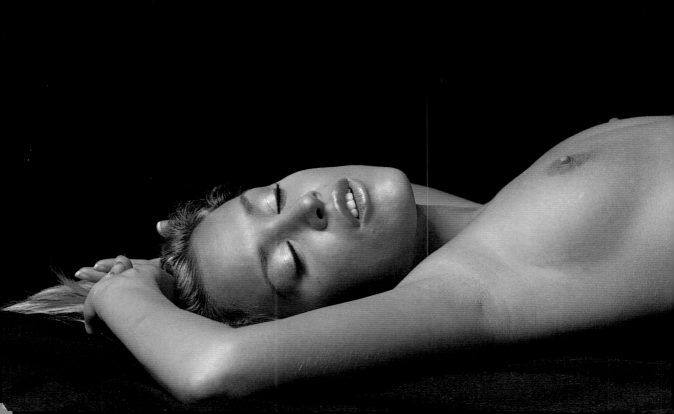

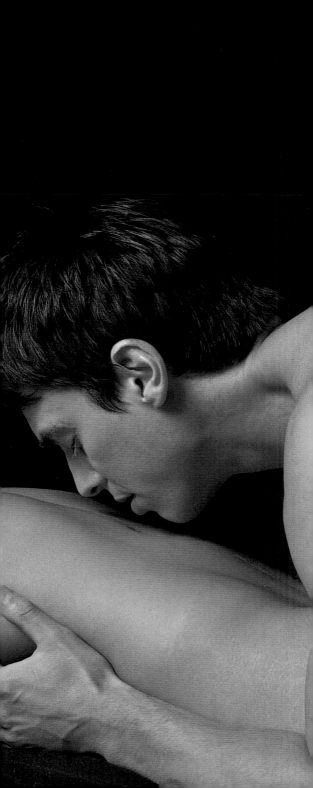

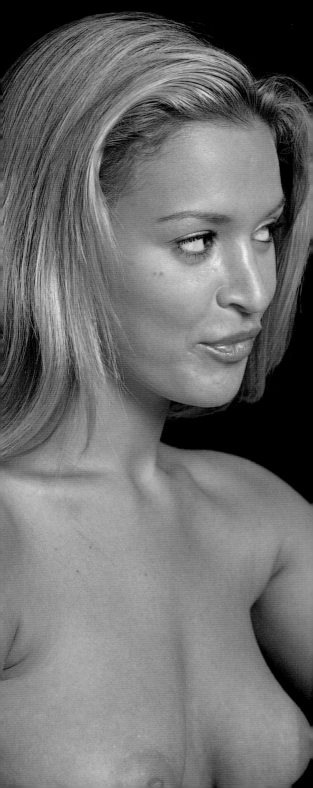

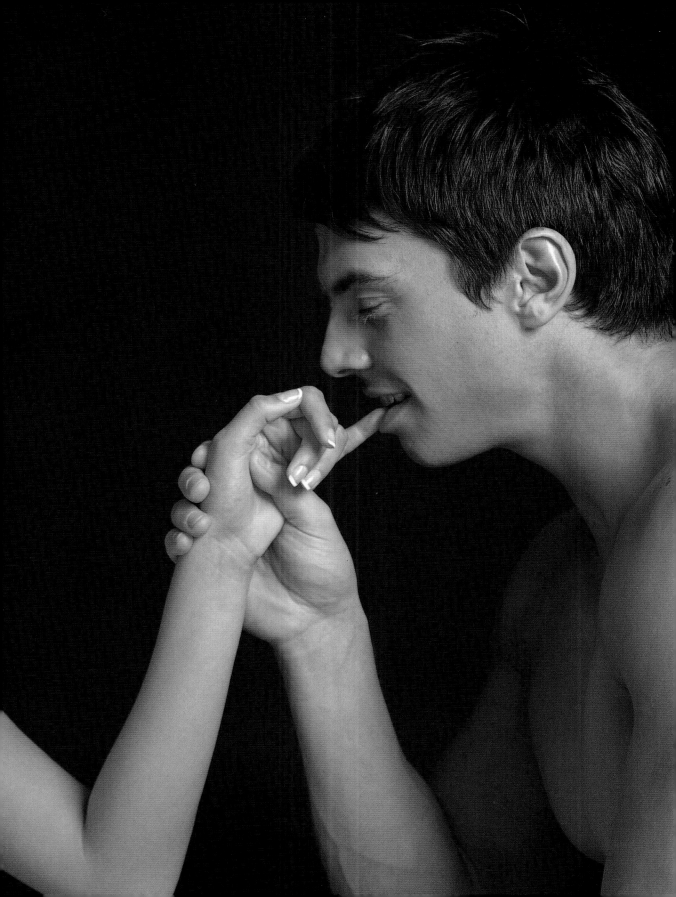

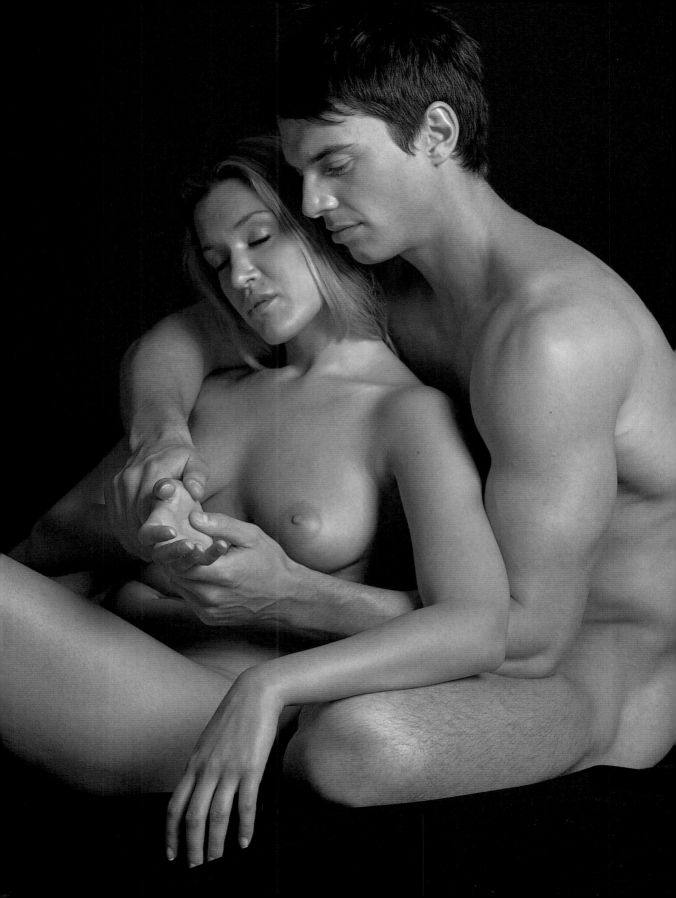

Back

Roll your partner over lovingly and massage his or her back with some oil using large, broad, gliding strokes. Find those tense areas at the top of the shoulders and lower neck and soothe away the knots. Do this while sitting astride your partner's body so that you grip him or her between your thighs, with your pubic hair and genital areas sliding over the buttocks and lower back whenever you move around to reach the highest parts of the back and neck.

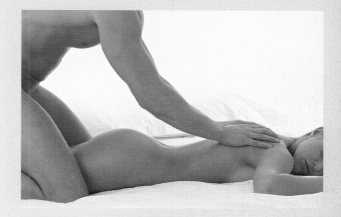

- Do some long gliding strokes up and down the large muscles at the sides of the spine, using your fingertips bunched together. Lose no opportunity to ensure the largest amount of skin contact between yourself and your partner.

Now lower your body position somewhat to get ready to do the buttocks. Sit between your partner's open legs as he or she lies on the front. This opens up the genital area and is in itself highly erotic.

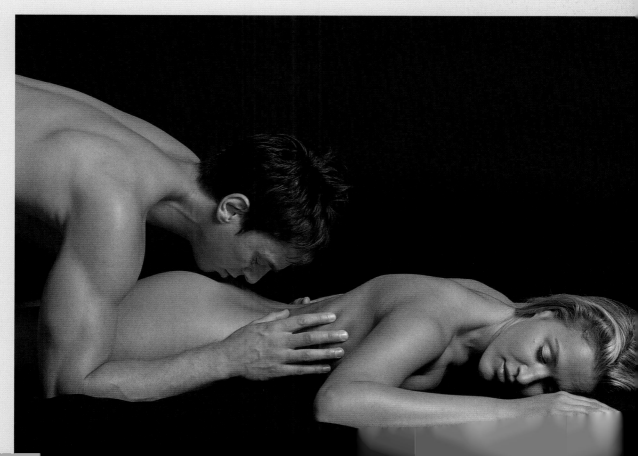

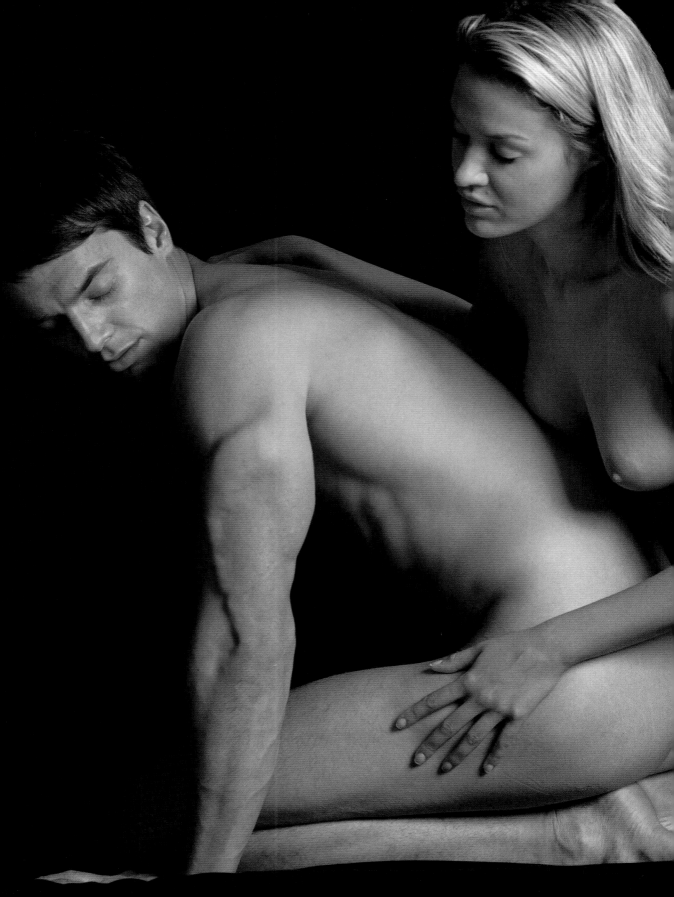

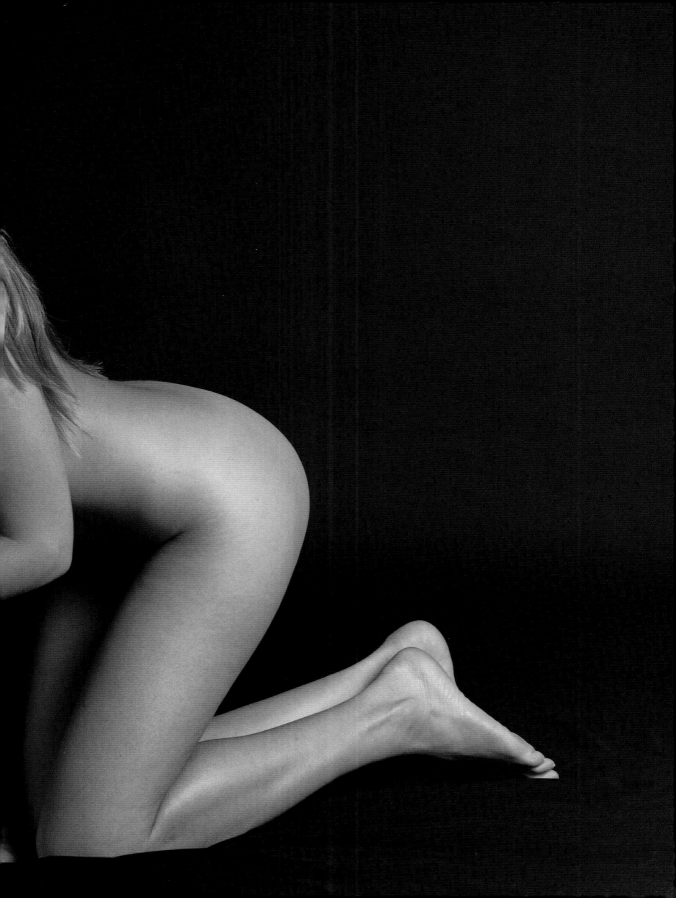

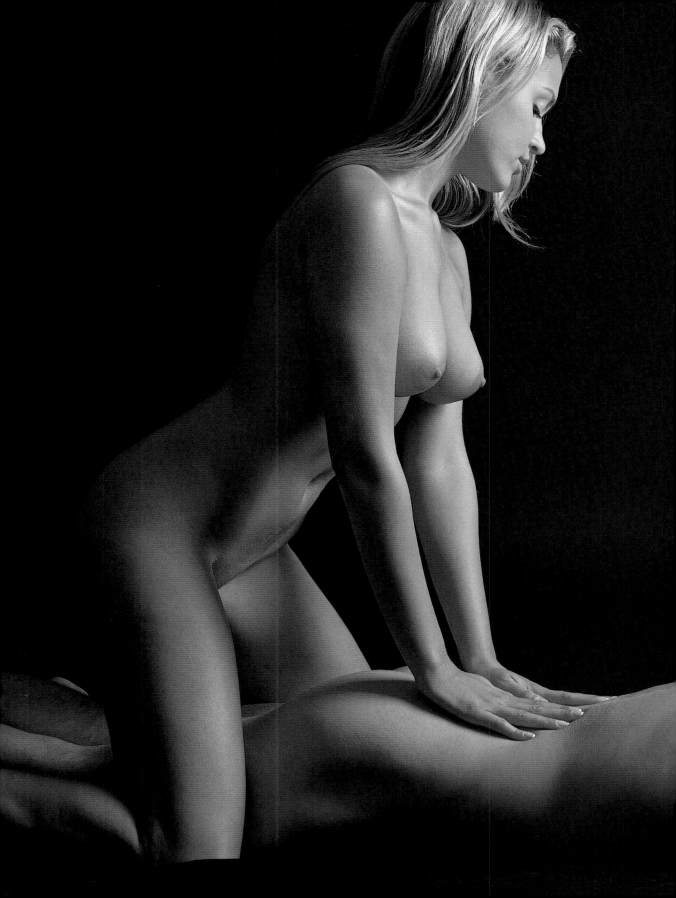

Buttocks

Many people greatly enjoy having their buttocks massaged and erotically stroked.

* Massage the buttocks and end up with teasing strokes down the crack between them.
* If your partner likes it, continue this stroke down to the anus and circle it in a teasing way.
* Massage the area between the anus and the vaginal opening or the base of the penis. This area—the perineum—is highly erogenous for most people yet is often totally ignored even by quite experienced couples.
* Do some long strokes from high up on the top of the spine—perhaps with your tongue—and continue on right down between the buttocks and then down to the anus or perineum. Make this journey long and highly erotic. Also be sure to make the endpoint worth waiting for.
* Massage the innermost parts of the buttocks but avoid the anus. Kiss the buttocks and run your hair all over them.

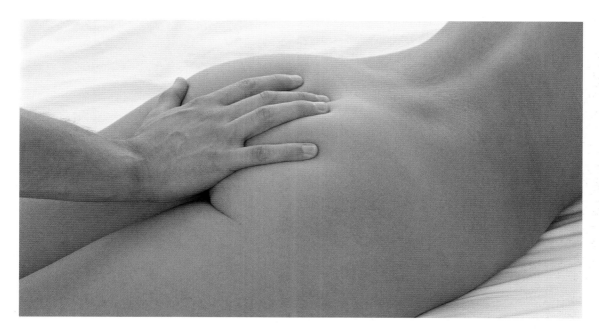

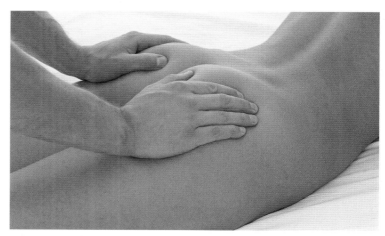

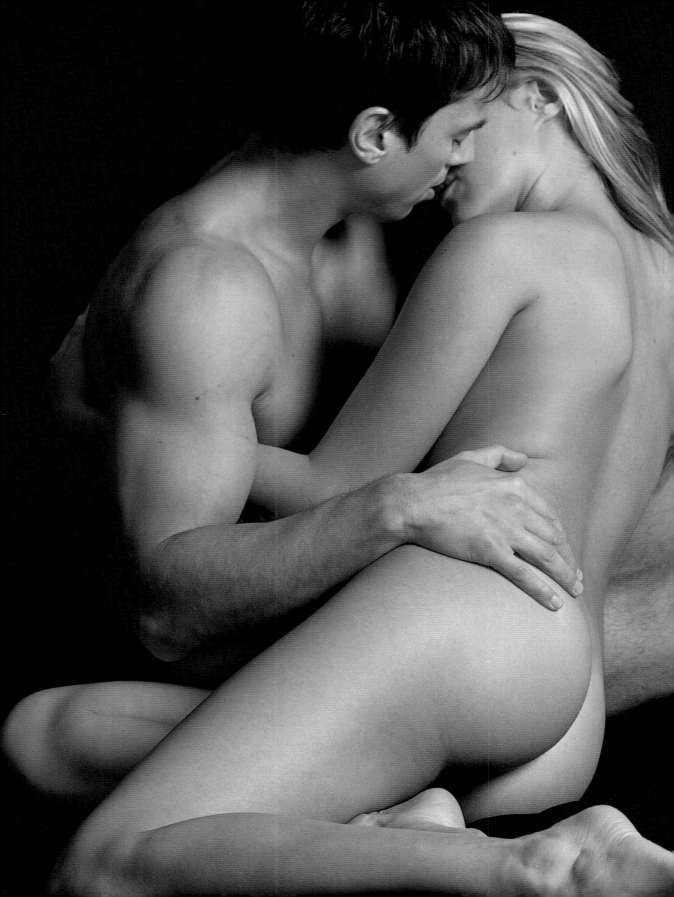

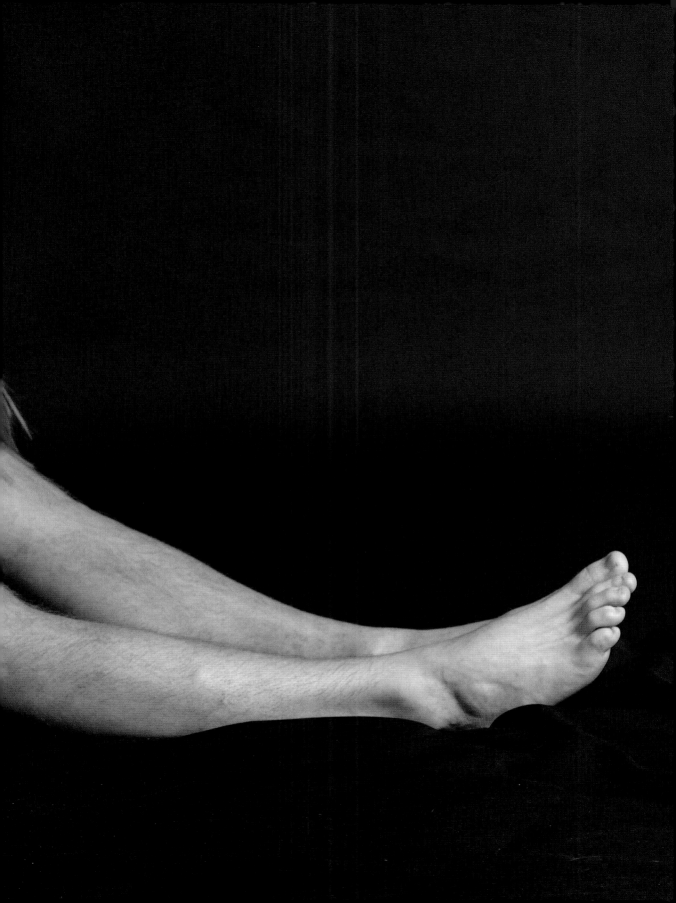

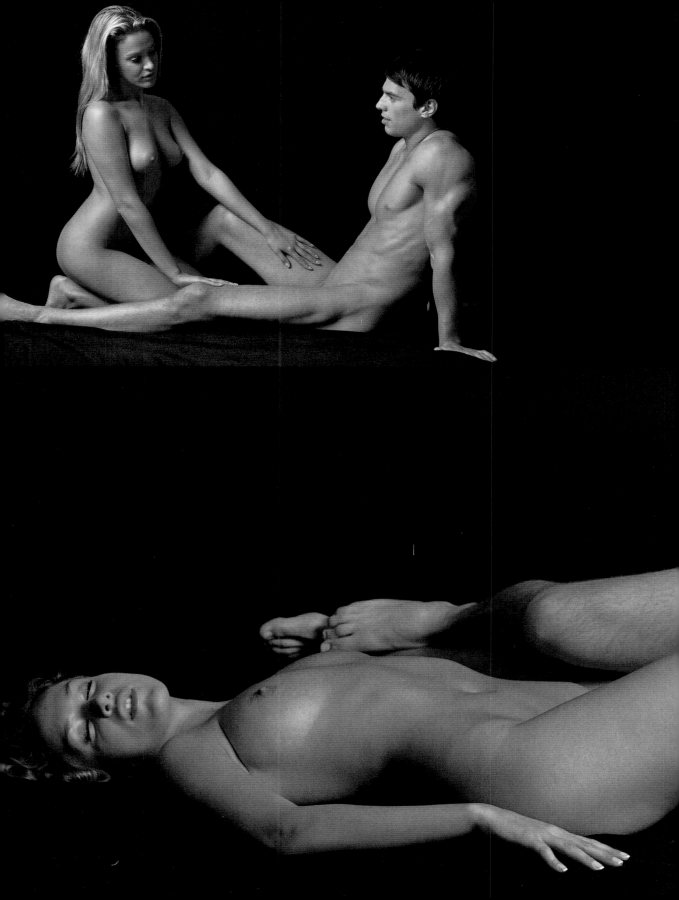

Legs and feet

Because the massage described so far has become so erotic the time has now come to slow the pace down a little:

- Smooth some oil onto your partner's legs and massage them, using long, gliding strokes from buttocks to ankles. Remember, as with the sensual massage, to put very little pressure on the skin as you go down and to be quite firm as you push up.
- The inner parts of the thighs are especially erotic for women, as are the areas behind the knees. Spend a lot of time massaging these areas and cover them with kisses and licks.

- Run your tongue right up to the pubic hair but do not actually touch it. Start behind the knee and with your tongue trace a path up to the genitals, via the inner thighs. Go back down again with your tongue and then cross to the other leg and repeat the process until he or she can bear it no more.
- Massage the feet as in the sensual massage section but this time use your mouth to kiss and enclose the toes and massage the feet themselves with parts of your body, including your genitals.
- Take your partner's foot and use it as if it were a massager to caress parts of your body you would like massaged and stroked.

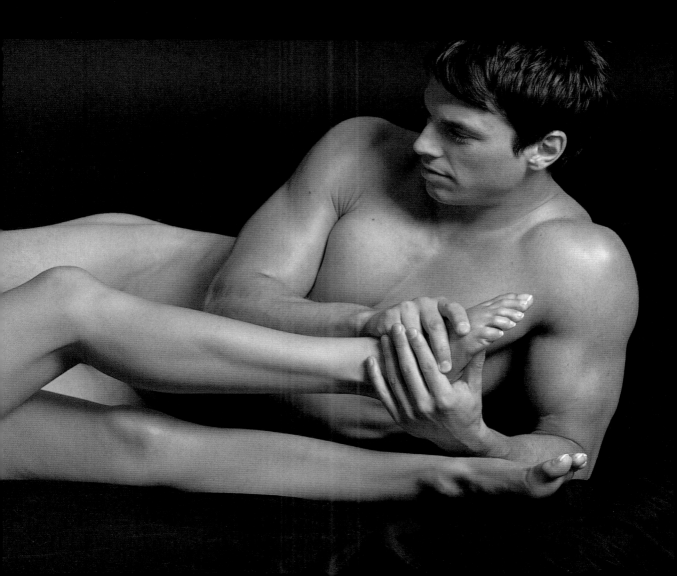

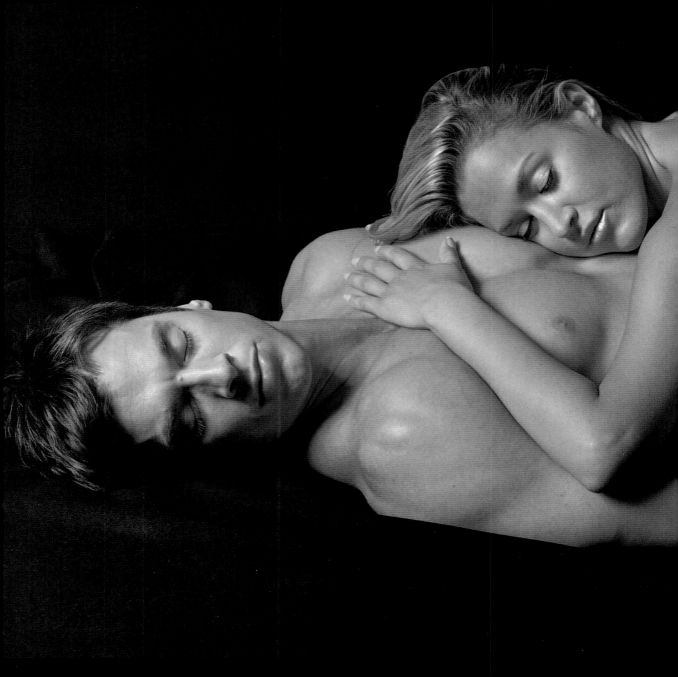

Whole body

Lastly, as with the sensual massage, but for different reasons, use your whole body to integrate all the areas you have been massaging so far. Rub yourself up and down various parts of his or her body, now using your genitals as additional massage aids. Go for long gliding strokes, first with you and then with your partner on top. Use various parts of your partner to massage yourself and generally luxuriate in the feel and warmth of one another's bodies.

By now you should be highly aroused and ready to start on more specifically genital play. How you do this is up to you and is beyond the scope of this book. Most couples who have taken their erotic massage this far will be so highly aroused that almost any genital activity will be exciting and orgasms should be rich, full and deeply satisfying.

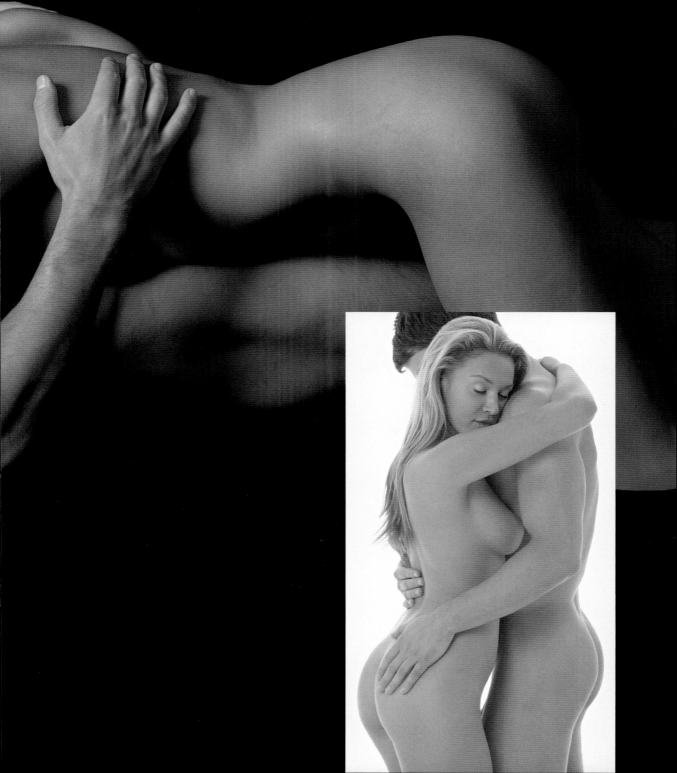

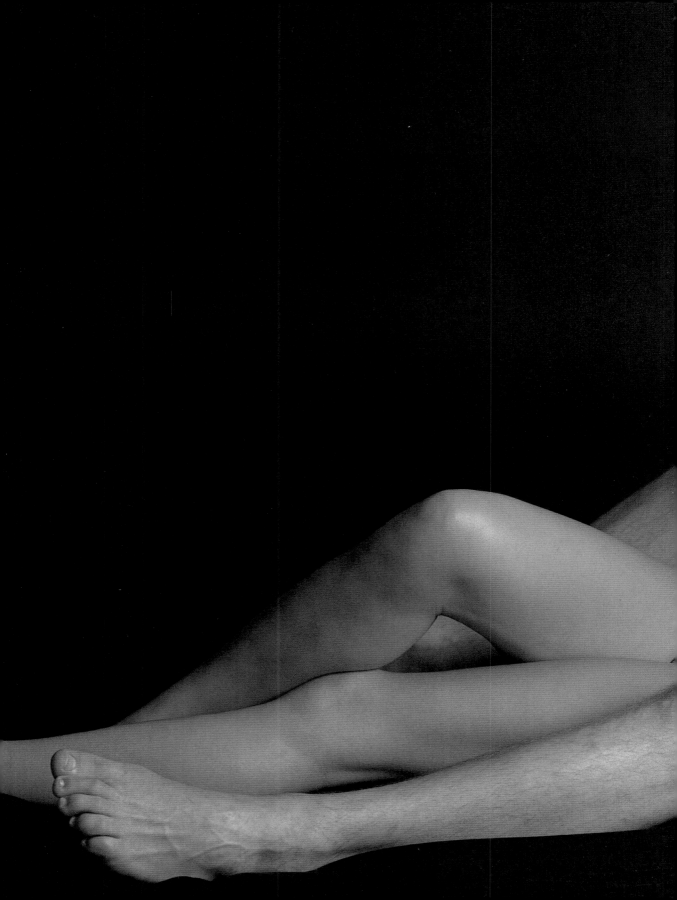

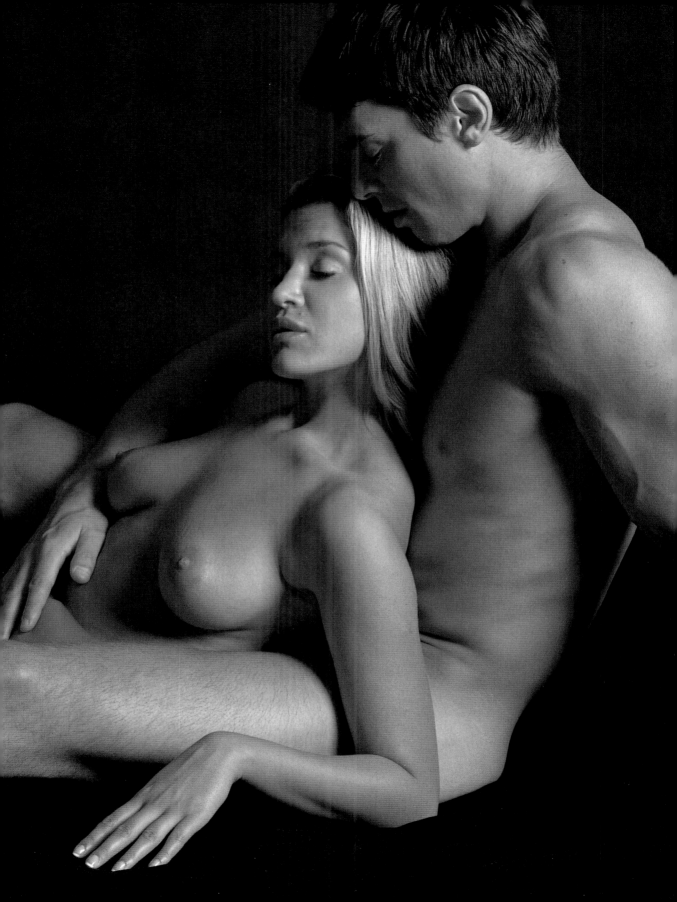

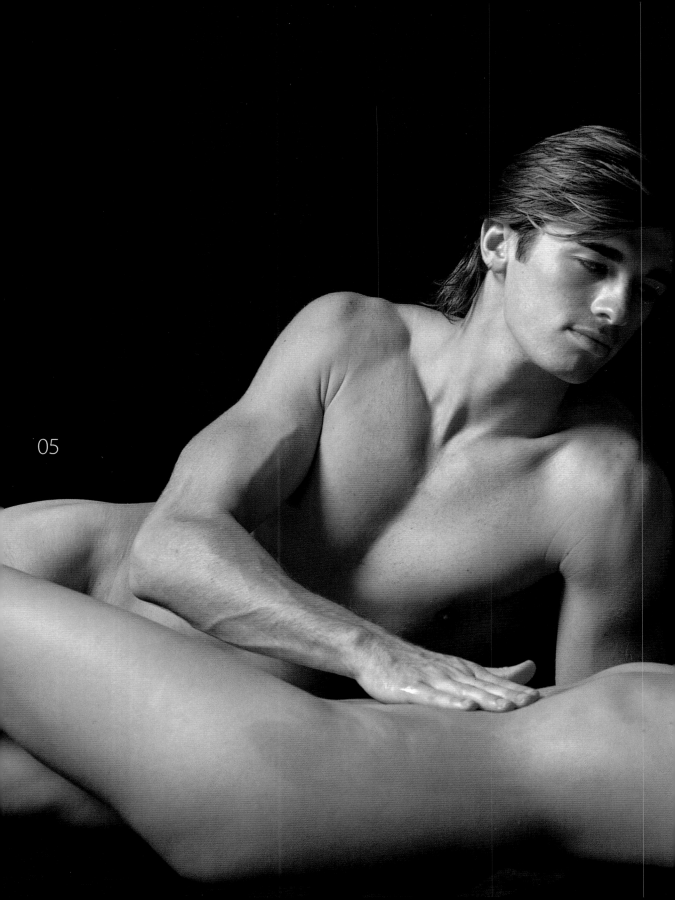

05

Natural therapies, massage, and sex

Although sex has many negative overtones in Western, Judeo-Christian culture, this is not so around the world and probably never has been.

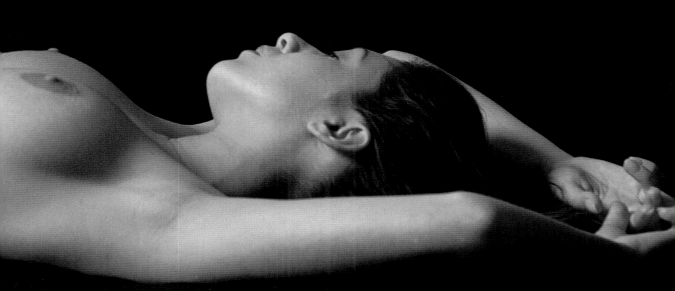

True, there have always been some prohibitions on sex (there are no cultures where anything goes with anybody at any time) but in the West we seem to have all kinds of hang-ups and inhibitions about sex.

Elsewhere in the world, on the contrary, sex is seen as an integral part of the splendor of life, and central to it. The ancient orientals placed sex on a high plane both in the universal scheme of things and for the individual. For them it fulfilled all kinds of spiritual roles as well as biological ones. Sadly, nowadays, the Western view of sexuality is fast taking over.

In my view this is a pity because sex is indeed a spiritual affair and the union between a couple who are lovers goes way beyond the physical embrace. Those readers who have this kind of relationship will know exactly what I mean.

In an increasingly harsh and godless world, I believe that for many the only glimpse of the spiritual world is to be found in their one-to-one relationship. In the absence of anything else, this is surely no bad thing.

What I perceive professionally is perfectly in keeping with this. As a marital therapist I see couples who function very well on the physical plane but certainly do not do so at the spiritual level. Their relationship is impoverished as a result, and they know it but do not know why.

All of these ideas become important when looking beyond the actual physical contact of sensual and erotic massage to the natural therapies, many of which are based on a wider understanding of the world than is the case in Western medicine. Indeed, the vast majority of such therapies have a vitally important spiritual dimension at their heart.

In this chapter I am looking very briefly at what some of the natural and often ancient massage therapies have to offer today's Western couple. While most readers will almost certainly use the sensual and erotic massage sections of the book on a day-to-day basis there are, I hope, some pleasant, relaxing and stimulating techniques in this chapter that could enrich almost any couple's experience. Few of us will be able to—or, indeed, even want to—embrace the philosophy or way of life that accompanies some of the therapies discussed but we can take from them techniques and skills that will help us to improve our sensual and erotic lives.

Aromatherapy This is an ancient art, dating back at least to the Pharaohs of Egypt, in which essential oils from plants are used medically to cure physical ailments or for their effects on the mind and the emotions. Occasionally the oils are taken internally but most often they are massaged into the skin, through which they are readily absorbed, especially if applied to skin which is warm after a bath.

As the oils are extracted from plants and flowers they can be expensive but a little goes a long way as they are very potent. Aromatherapy oils are widely available and at good prices. Buy the best ones you can afford, bearing in mind that you'll be able to dilute the neat oil with a much cheaper carrier oil. A few drops of neat oil are all you need in one tablespoon of vegetable oil. Of course, if you want to you can buy specially prepared aromatherapy massage oils but they are more expensive.

Aromatherapy is easy to practice at home because all you need is the oil and your hands. We shall not consider the therapeutic use of aromatherapy oils here because this is something that should be done only by a professional, but we shall look at their use as part of sensual and erotic massage. In this context the best way to choose which oil to use is to see which scent you prefer.

If you like the smell of a particular oil, it will probably have a relaxing effect on you as its "odoriferous molecules"—the active ingredients that create the smell—act on your brain via your nostrils. Smell is a very primitive and highly developed sensory system in all animals, and humans are no exception.

Once you have bought your oil it can be used a few drops at a time in the bath. You can also put three or four drops into a bowl of hot water to inhale; or you can use it to massage yourself or your partner.

Unless you have bought an aromatherapy oil that is ready for use straight from the bottle, it is cheaper and perfectly effective to dilute it with a carrier oil such as soy or almond oil; use three or four drops of oil to one eggcupful of the carrier oil.

To enhance the effects of the oil, the receiver's skin should first be warmed either by massaging him

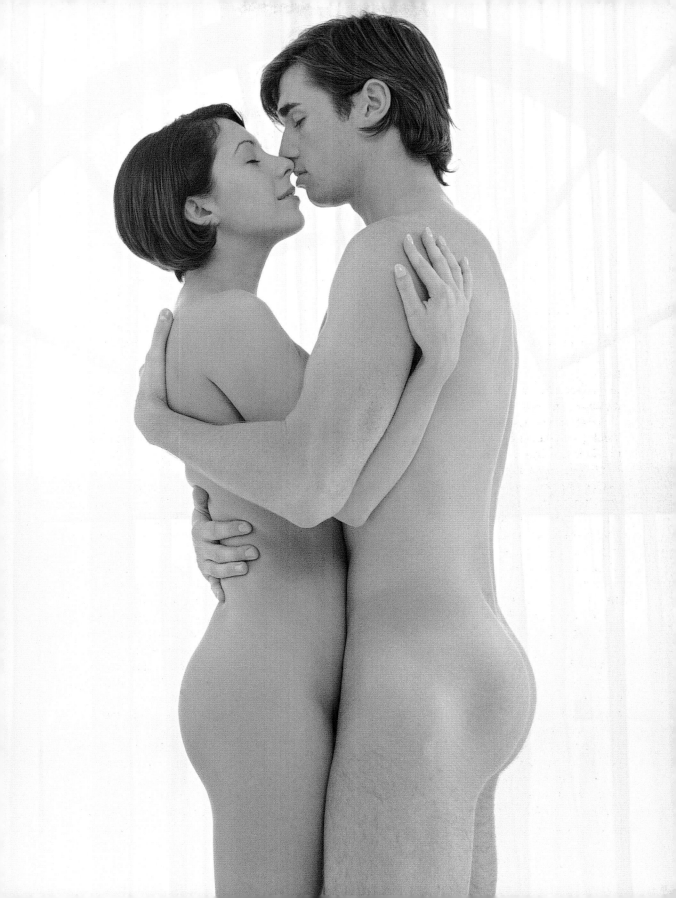

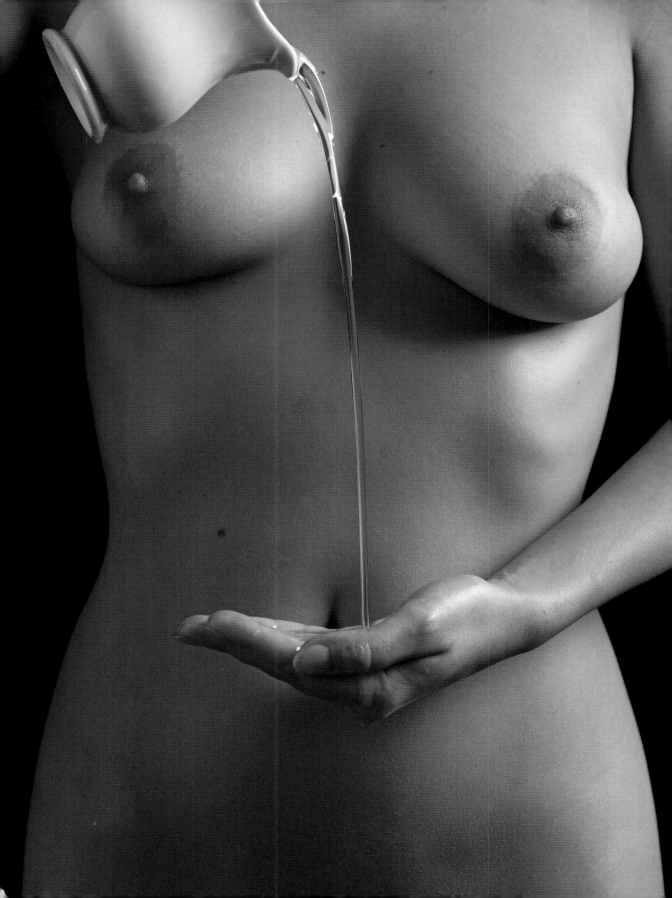

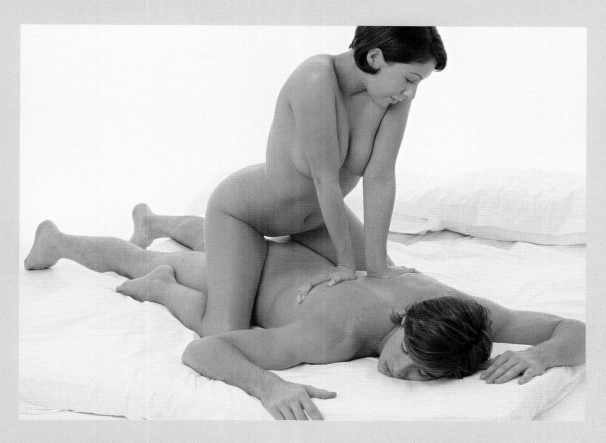

or her without oil or by using it after he or she has had a bath or shower. Use the oil to massage your partner as discussed throughout the book. The difference between using ordinary massage oil and aromatherapy oils is that the exquisite scent of the latter will have effects of its own which will add to the relaxing or erotic effects of the massage itself.

Here are a few notes on particular aromatherapy oils and their uses in conditions that might be of interest to you as you learn to use these oils as part of your sensual and erotic life together.

Rosemary oil is said to have an aphrodisiac effect. Add four drops to a tablespoon of soy oil, mix well and massage into the area around the base of the spine.

Caraway oil added to the bath has been found to help ease period pains.

Sage oil, 3 drops to a bowl of warm water or bidet and splashed up into the vagina helps cure infections and soothe irritations.

Peppermint can be used as a gargle, in a dose of 2 drops to a cup or glassful of warm water. This is repeated when necessary as a cure for unpleasant-smelling breath.

Using aromatherapy oils is unlikely to become a regular part of your massage routine on the grounds of cost but for those special occasions when you want to enhance the mood or feel particularly relaxed, they can be quite magical.

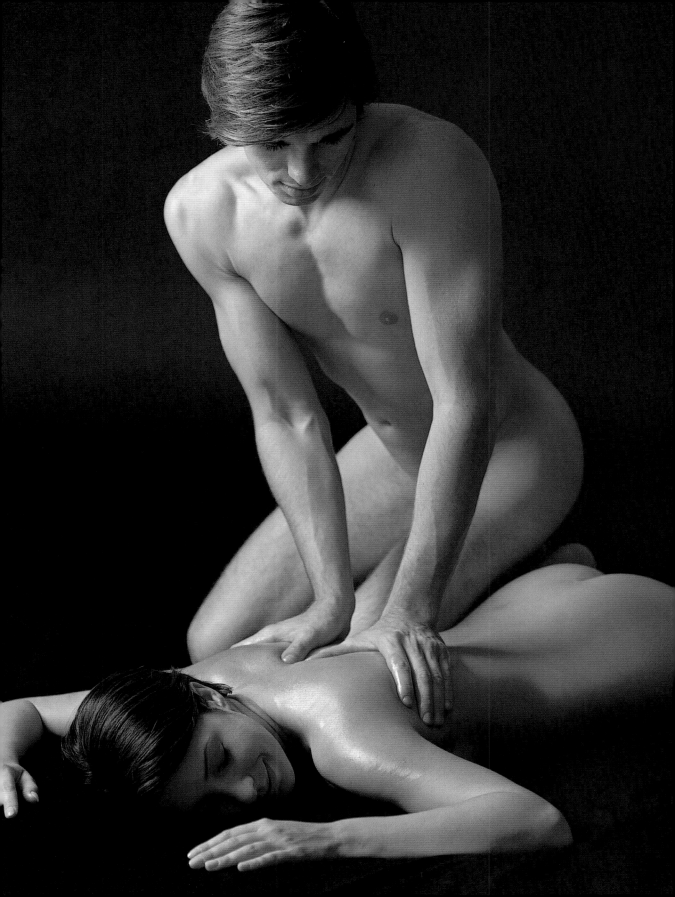

Shiatsu
This literally means "finger pressure" and is an ancient Japanese art. It is different from Western forms of massage in that it uses only pressure and stretching strokes.

The practitioner of Shiatsu uses fingers, elbows, knees or feet to work on the many acupuncture points along the body's energy channels. It is rather like the closely related art of Chinese acupressure but this latter uses only fingers to apply pressure.

Although much of Western massage is in fact aimed at balancing the body's energy patterns and flows, we do not usually talk of things in this way, whereas Shiatsu confronts this head-on.

As you would imagine, it is a lifetime's task to become truly expert at Shiatsu but there is much that the amateur can achieve at home with a little practice. As with all the forms of massage I have discussed, the results largely depend on the level of communication between the giver and the receiver. Posture is important when practicing Shiatsu. Both giver and receiver should be relaxed and when you apply the pressure to an acupuncture point it should all come from the area just below your navel (the *hara*) rather than from your arms or shoulders. It is also important to press on the pressure points (*tsubos*) with your thumb or palm at right angles to your body.

Kneel with your legs slightly apart so that you feel steady and firm. This will enable you to sustain the pressure over some time without losing your balance or becoming tired. Keep your arms straight. Ideally, the receiver should be on the floor, but if the relevant *tsubos* can be easily reached with the receiver sitting in a chair, that is fine.

Although the true professional uses many parts of his body to apply pressure, it is easiest for the beginner to start with his or her thumbs. Apply pressure with one thumb only, though at times both will need to be used, one on top of the other. Use the pad of your thumb and allow the rest of your hand to lie on the receiver's body to maintain contact. In fact, always keep your hands in contact with your partner's body; if necessary use one hand to apply the pressure and allow the other to rest on the body close to your working hand.

You can also use your palm to press over the person's *hara*; press with your arm at right angles to the receiver's body.

Pressure during a shiatsu massage usually feels pleasant and comfortable to the receiver but if ever he or she feels pain or discomfort, stop, because this may suggest internal problems.

The receiver need not be naked for this type of massage but it is probably better if he or she is.

Before describing a brief massage sequence that can be used by anyone who has some experience of sensual massage, it makes sense to think for a moment about times when it is unwise to do such a massage.

- Beware especially of varicose veins.
- Avoid the abdomen of a pregnant woman and, in later stages of pregnancy, avoid pressure on the legs.
- Do not massage anyone who is exhausted.
- Don't massage anyone with a fever.
- Do not massage anyone with a contagious skin disease, a slipped disc, or broken bones.

Anyone who really wants to learn about performing a good shiatsu massage must do the appropriate research. Here, though, is a brief résumé of a simple shiatsu massage that will integrate your partner's energy systems and enhance his or her sense of well-being. Remember that all of these strokes act on various acupuncture points in such a way as to alter and to normalize energy flows in them.

Ask your partner to lie on his or her stomach, flat on the floor or mat. Place your hands diagonally across the back, over one shoulder blade and the opposite hip and stretch the spine as the receiver breathes out. Change over your hands and repeat the stretch across the other dimension of the back.

Press along the top of each shoulder and rotate the shoulder blades. Here there are meridians (energy flow channels) that have to do with tension and stress. Use your thumbs, elbows and even the heels of your feet to apply pressure here.

Apply pressure all along both sides of the spine. Do this first with your palms then with your thumbs.

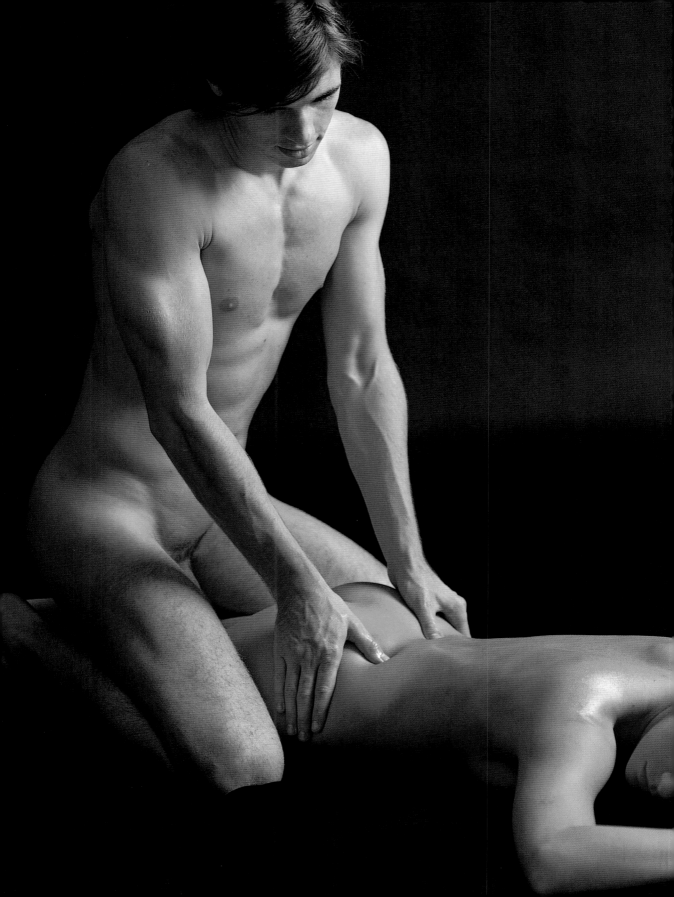

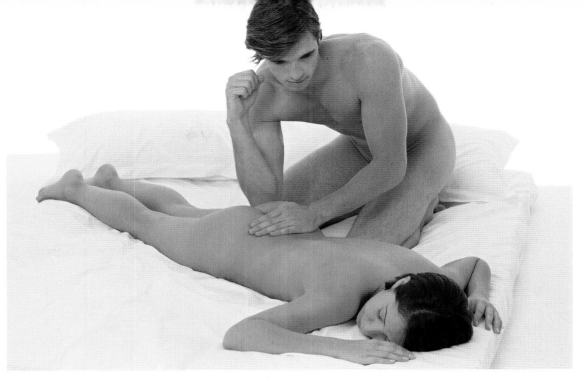

Next, go to the hips and use your thumbs to press over the sacrum (the lowest part of the back where it joins the bottom) as shown on the opposite page. Squeeze the sides of the buttocks and then use your elbow to knead the upper curve of the buttocks.

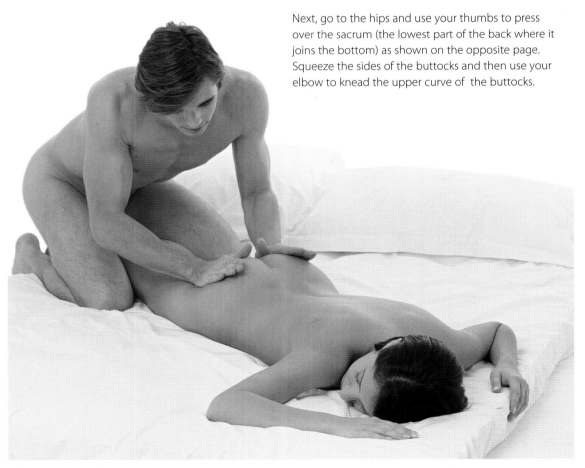

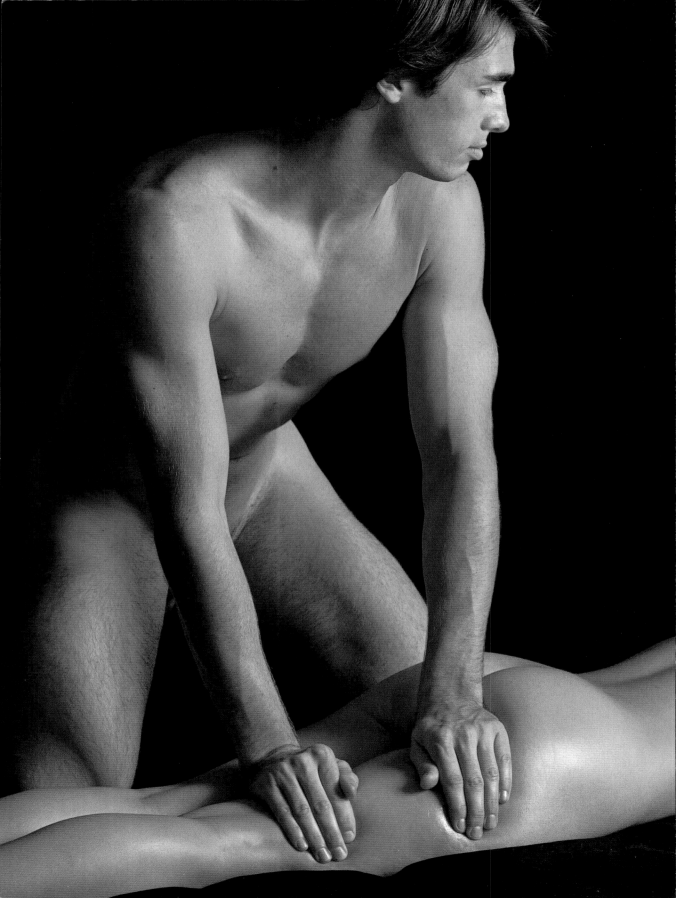

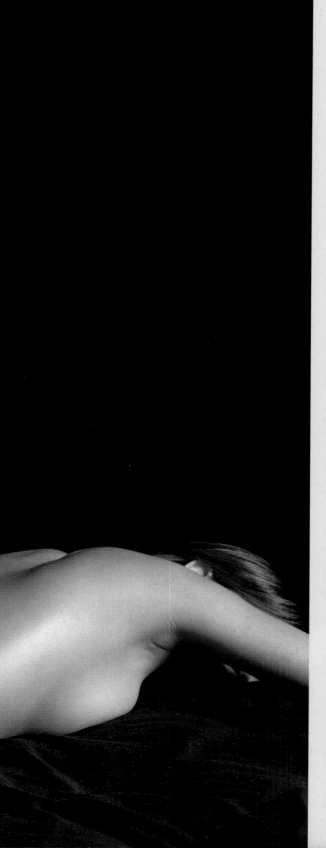

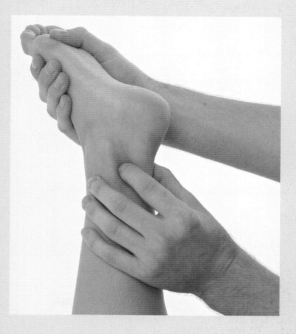

Now work down the center of the back of each leg, first with your palm and then your knees. Press lightly at the side of the Achilles tendon for about 3 to 5 seconds.

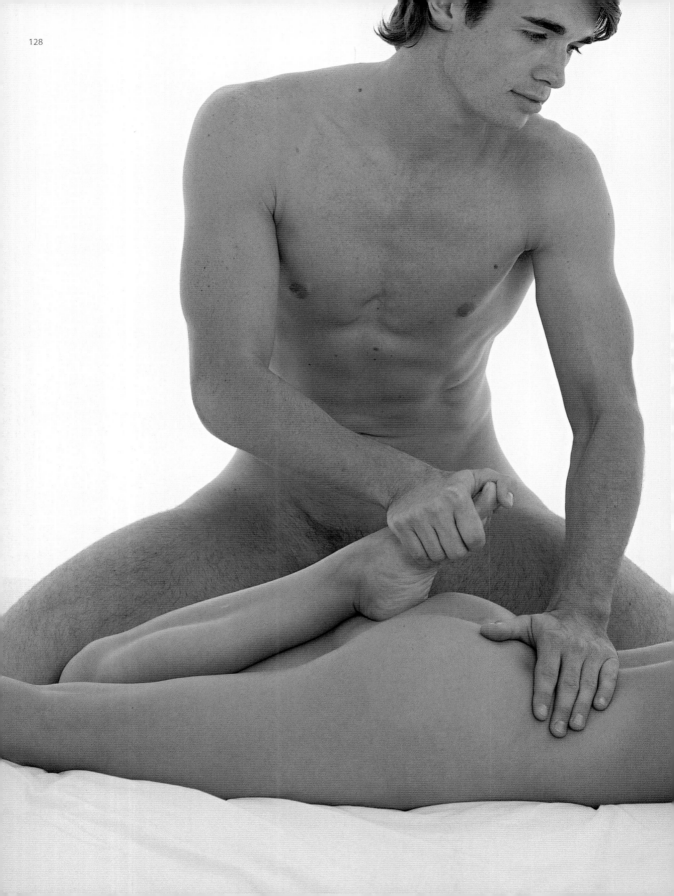

Stretch the leg by placing one hand on the small of the back and carefully bringing the foot back toward the buttock, holding the foot under the toes for the best stretch. If the receiver shows any sign of discomfort stop at once. Next put your partner's leg at right angles to the body and press firmly down with both palms on the top surface.

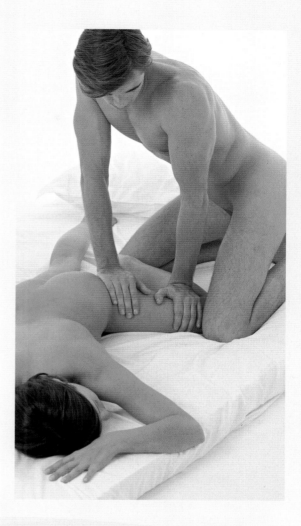

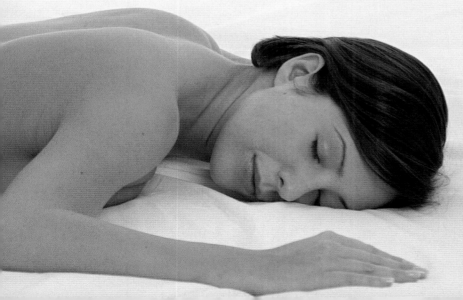

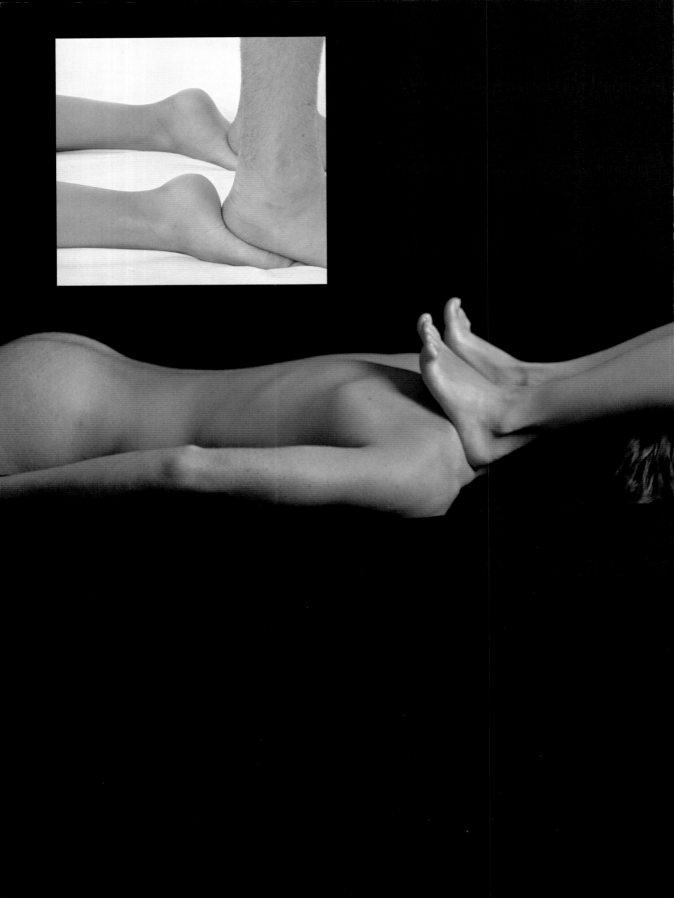

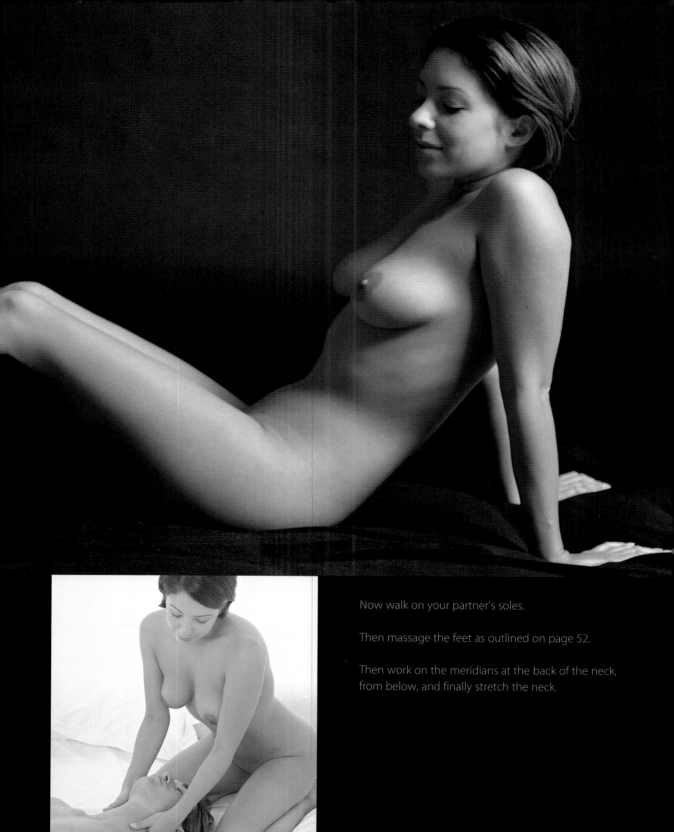

Now walk on your partner's soles.

Then massage the feet as outlined on page 52.

Then work on the meridians at the back of the neck, from below, and finally stretch the neck.

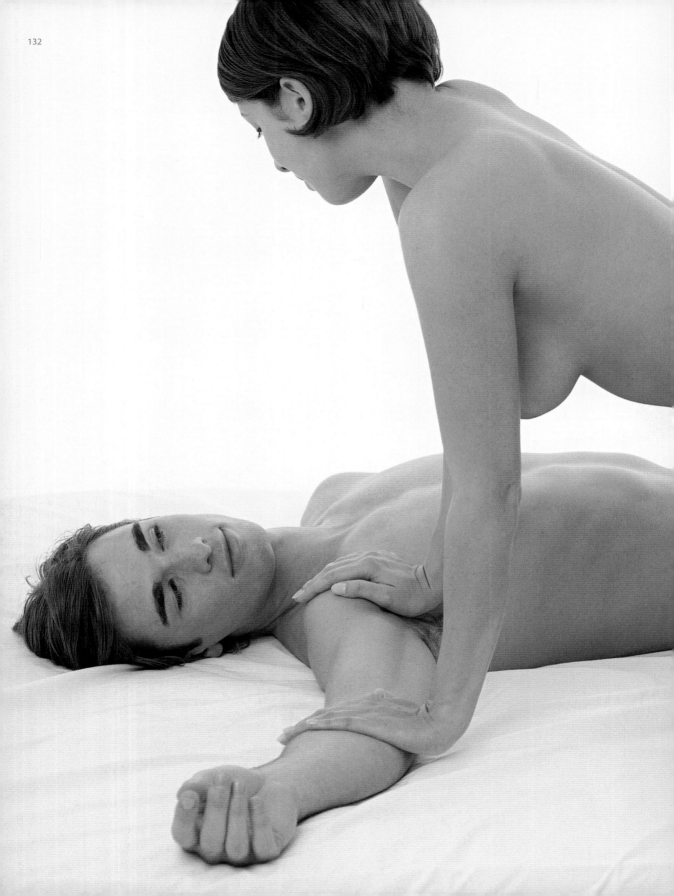

Work around the face as described on page 42.

Turn next to the arms, applying palm pressure along each inner arm in turn with your partner's palm upward.

Apply palm pressure down the forearm, with his or her palm facing downward.

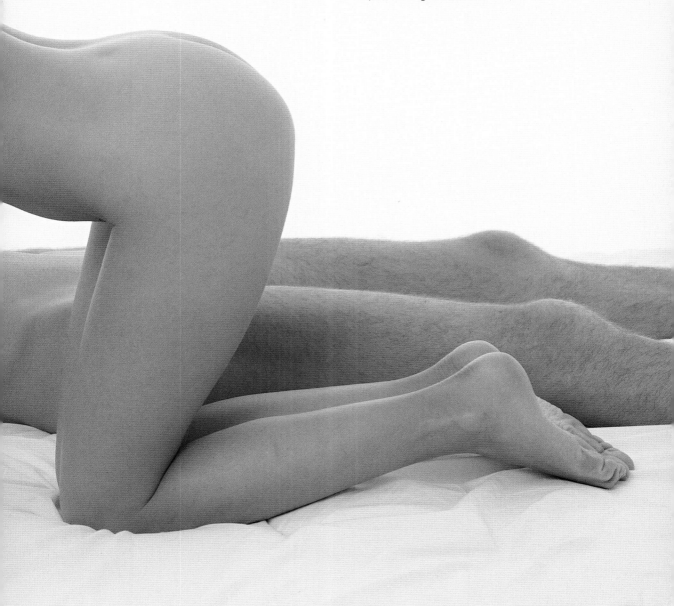

Then turn your attention to the hands. Pull the fingers gently before going on to stimulate the area in the web between the thumb and the first finger. Press here for 5 seconds using your fingers on the palm side and your thumb on the top of his or her hand.

Now take hold of your partner's hand at the wrist and gently shake the arm to loosen and relax it.

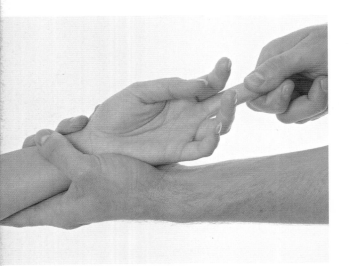

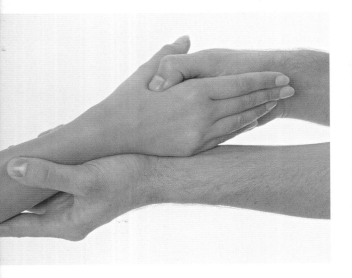

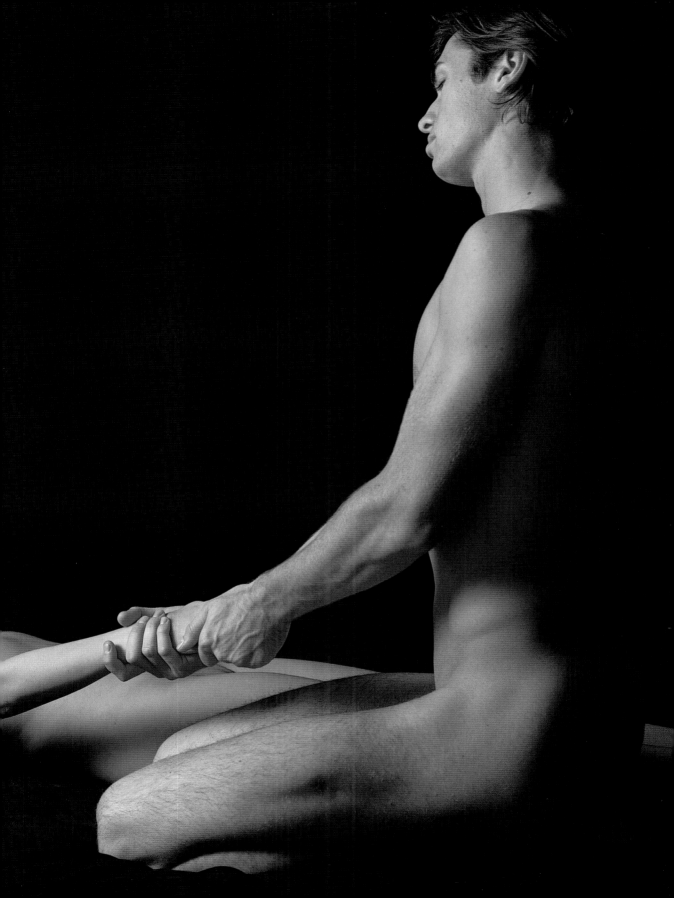

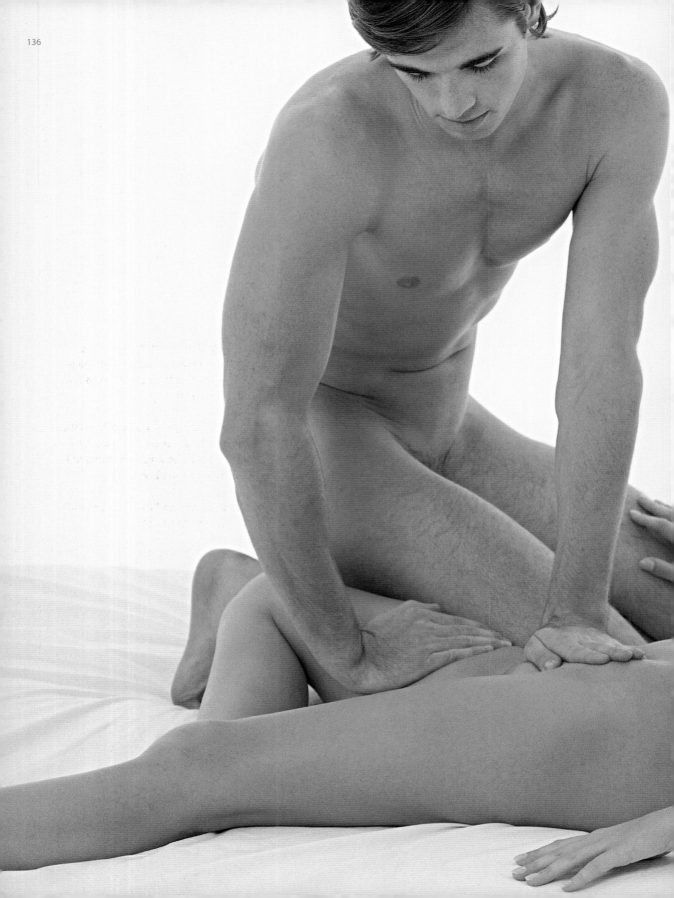

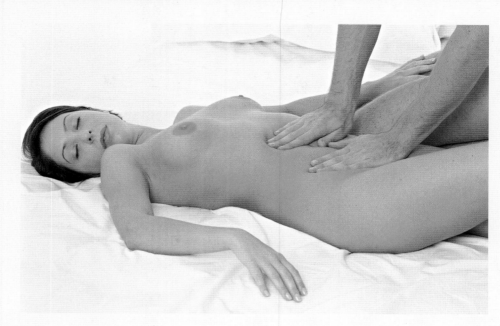

Massage the lower area of the stomach—the *hara*. Work around the area clockwise, as outlined on page 49, then press gently under both sides of the ribs and down the midline to the navel.

Complete your shiatsu massage by working down the fronts of the legs with palm pressure, first down the inside of the thigh and lower leg and then down the outside, avoiding pressure on the bone.

Stretch the foot first backward and then forward and repeat the whole sequence on the other leg.

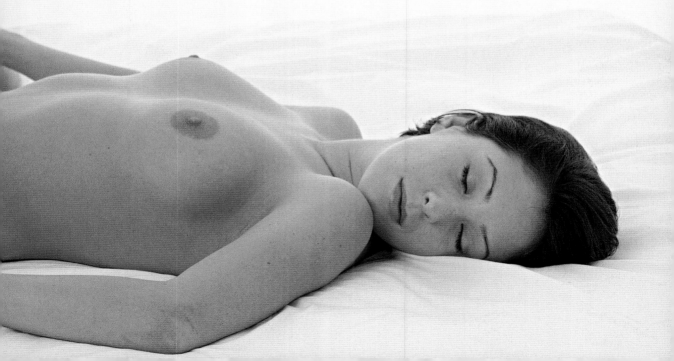

I must stress that this kind of shiatsu is a simple do-it-yourself, relaxing, pleasure-centered pursuit. It is not supposed to be directly "healing" for any specific condition. It is safest to go to a professional therapist if you are searching for a cure of any kind.

Having said this, the rather different techniques involved here can be a pleasant change and can often have more profound mental and emotional effects than an ordinary sensual massage. In fact, some people find that, if it is done properly, a shiatsu massage can be very moving and can mobilize all kinds of emotions. It is vital therefore, that the person doing the giving can be trusted by the receiver. It is difficult or near impossible to relax completely and allow oneself to become totally vulnerable to one's feelings if one fears being let down, criticized, ridiculed, or ignored if emotions begin to surface.

As with all forms of massage, the main elements are understanding, love, trust and care, and the best massage experiences result from this empathy coming across to the receiver.

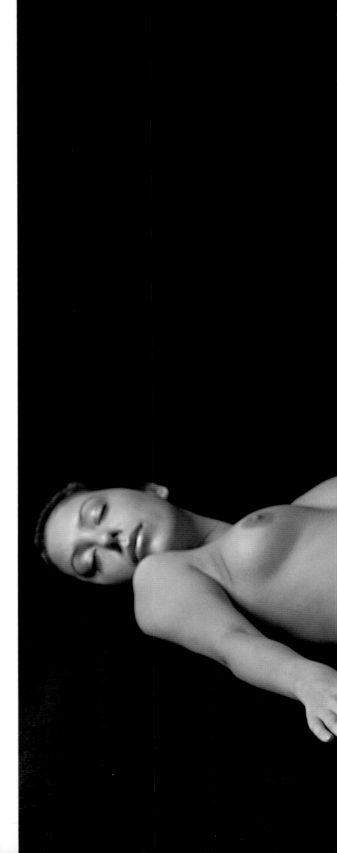

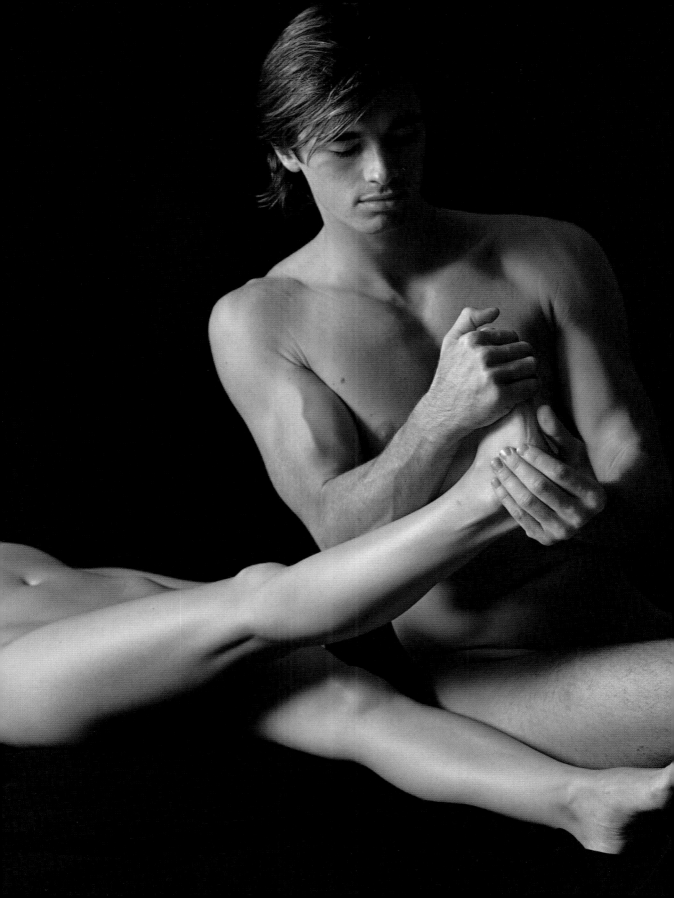

Acupressure

This is closely related to shiatsu, and there is little doubt that the correct stimulation of certain acupuncture points has a beneficial effect on the body, mind, and spirit generally. Although no amateur massage enthusiast will ever become familiar enough with the acupuncture points to treat illnesses in any meaningful way, some of the points are easy to find and to apply pressure to, often with excellent results.

You simply use thumb pressure over the known acupuncture points to produce both local and distant effects on the body. Here are some suggestions. Press each point for about 4 seconds, two or three times.

Back
- Each side of the spine
- Along the shoulder ridge

Hips
- Sides of the buttocks
- Over the sacrum
- Center of the buttock crease

Ankles
- Both sides of the Achilles tendon simultaneously

Feet
- Center of the ball of foot
- One or two inches above the skin connecting the big toe and second toe

Shoulders
- An inch or two below the hollow at the outer end of the collarbone

Arms and Hands
- In the web between the thumb and first finger

Hara
- Three inches to either side of the navel (press in toward navel)

- Press with the flats of four fingers, two inches below the navel, centrally

Legs
- Back of each knee
- Top of shinbone, as in the illustration. Press hard. If you are on the correct point, a powerful sensation will run down to the ankle.

Pressure on these points often adds a special dimension to what would otherwise have been an ordinary, if pleasant, massage, and pressing over all of these areas is safe in healthy people, except for the area between the thumb and first finger, which should not be pressed in pregnant women.

If pressure anywhere causes pain or discomfort, however, stop at once and discuss the matter with an acupuncturist. You may simply have pressed too hard but it is always better not to make such assumptions.

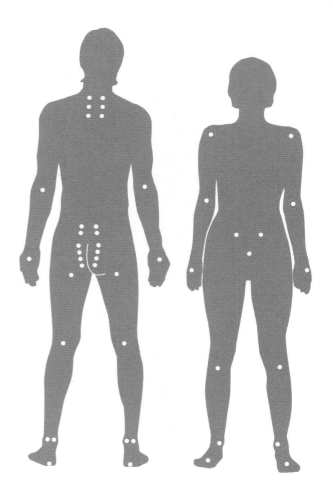

Reflexology

Reflexology works on the basis that there are reflex zones in the soles of the feet corresponding to every part of the body. It is claimed that pressure and manipulation of these areas harmonize the energy flows in the body and make the receiver feel relaxed.

Learning reflexology is best done at a proper seminar or course and a book such as this is no place to go into any detail. Suffice it to say that massaging the feet can be very relaxing, if you follow certain basic tips.

The finger and thumb techniques of reflexology are rather different from normal massage and they really should be learned from an expert.

Do not attempt this kind of massage on pregnant women or anyone with severe varicose veins or phlebitis.

However, it is possible to massage the feet by using a simple reflexology technique. The best position for this is to have the receiver sitting in a reclining chair or in an ordinary, comfortable chair with his feet up on a stool, at the same level as your lap.

Oil is not the best lubricant for this kind of massage. Instead, try talcum powder or even cornflour. Place a towel on your lap and massage one foot at a time.

Now take one forefoot and, sandwiching it between your hands, move the front half of the foot backward and forward. Then support the heel of the foot in one hand while you rotate the front of the foot with the other.

To work on the whole foot, grasp the toes with your thumb on the big toe and your other fingers holding the receiver's other toes. This fixes the foot and slightly stretches the sole. Now take the thumb of the hand you intend to use and bend it at the first joint to barely a

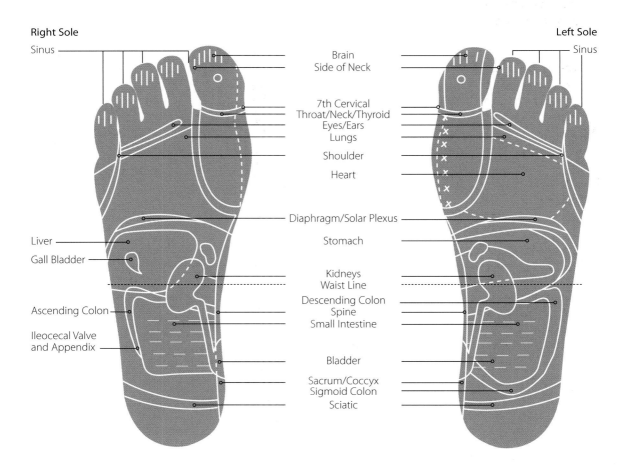

Right Sole

Sinus
Liver
Gall Bladder
Ascending Colon
Ileocecal Valve and Appendix

Brain
Side of Neck
7th Cervical
Throat/Neck/Thyroid
Eyes/Ears
Lungs
Shoulder
Heart
Diaphragm/Solar Plexus
Stomach
Kidneys
Waist Line
Descending Colon
Spine
Small Intestine
Bladder
Sacrum/Coccyx
Sigmoid Colon
Sciatic

Left Sole

Sinus

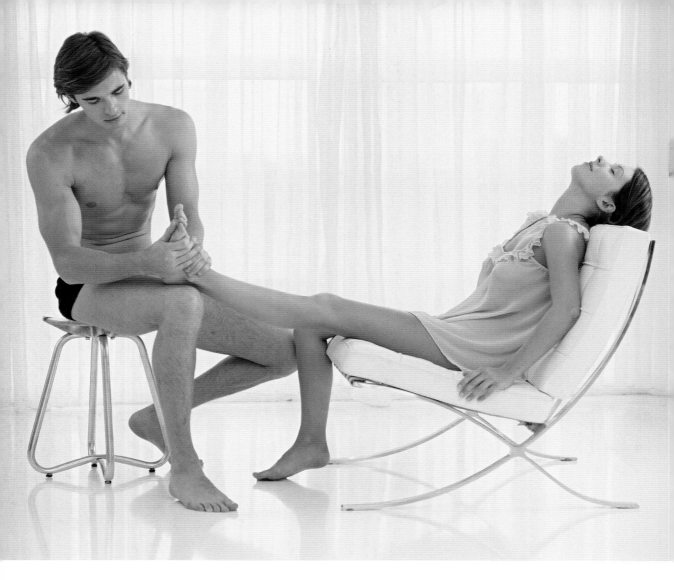

right angle. Place the tip of this bent thumb on the sole of the receiver's foot and, working the bent joint, "walk" your thumb along the foot. The receiver should not feel your nail if you have your thumb in the correct position. For the best possible results, the inside edge of your thumb should be the area that is in contact with the various zones of the foot (nor the actual tip). Because the reflex points are located under the skin quite deep pressure is needed to affect them.

It is not wise to massage the feet in this way if someone is unwell. However, for a relaxing and toning treatment you can start at the toes and slowly work your way down to the heels after studying the layout of the main reflex zones in the diagram. When you have completed massaging the sole, begin work on the sides of the feet.

As you walk your thumb over the skin, be careful if you come to any areas of tenderness or grittiness because if you press too hard here the individual will be tensed rather than relaxed.

End by holding the foot and rotating it, as you did when you started, then briefly hold the foot between both of your hands. Repeat the whole process on the other foot.

If you have done this well, your partner will be very relaxed. This is a very pleasant way to relax a friend whom you do not know sufficiently well to do a whole body massage on.

Some people enjoy receiving a hand massage performed in much the same way. This, too, works on the principle that parts of the body are represented in the reflex zones of the hands.

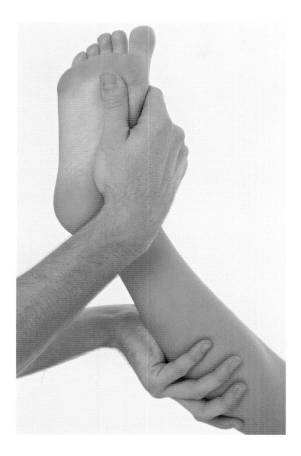

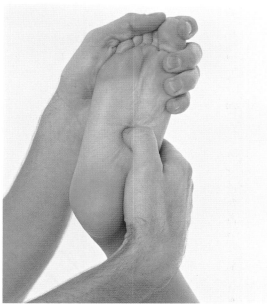

In conclusion Although none of the "alternative" massage methods I have briefly outlined in this section are erotic in themselves, many couples find them either stimulating or relaxing and this can be the starting point for an erotic massage. An individual whose feet have just been massaged using reflexology techniques or someone who has had their acupuncture points massaged systematically might well feel so relaxed that they want to have sex, perhaps after some erotic massage.

But as I have stressed throughout the book, all of these methods—apart, of course, from erotic massage itself—should be seen simply as "gifts" from the giver to the receiver. Unless a couple agree beforehand that sex is to be the endpoint, it is far better to leave things to take their course and see what happens as the session progresses. Some people start off just asking for their feet to be massaged, for example, and begin to feel not only extremely relaxed but even sexually aroused.

It is important to remember that, whatever we do with our partner, it should be the joy of giving that lies at the heart of any good massage. But this needs to be matched by the receiver being at one with the giver, in tune with his or her efforts so that the massage time is rewarding for both. This leads to communication, both verbal and nonverbal, at the time of the massage, or afterward. Such two-way communication is central to all massage, of whatever kind, and it is this that makes massage so magical a pursuit for many couples.

In an age of goal-centered sex and worries about sexual performance this giving and receiving of one another freely is arguably one of the most priceless gifts in a loving relationship.

Index